前　言

《循证针灸临床实践指南》包括：带状疱疹、贝尔面瘫、抑郁症、中风后假性球麻痹、偏头痛、颈椎病、慢性便秘、腰痛、原发性痛经、坐骨神经痛、失眠、成人支气管哮喘、肩周炎、膝关节炎、急慢性胃炎、过敏性鼻炎、突发性耳聋、三叉神经痛、糖尿病周围神经病变、单纯性肥胖病等病症的循证针灸临床实践指南。

本部分为《循证针灸临床实践指南》的中风后假性球麻痹部分。

本部分受国家中医药管理局指导与委托。

本部分由中国针灸学会提出。

本部分由中国针灸学会标准化工作委员会归口。

本部分起草单位：北京中医药大学东直门医院、中国中医科学院针灸研究所。

本部分主要起草人：赵吉平、王军、李俊、白鹏、王鹏、郭盛楠、陈晟、赵宏、武晓冬、訾明杰、郭旭。

本部分专家组成员：刘保延、房繁恭、刘志顺、吴泰相、吴中朝、杨金洪、梁繁荣、张维、刘炜宏、杨金生、文碧玲、余曙光、郭义、杨骏、赵京生、杨华元、储浩然、石现、王富春、王麟鹏、贾春生、余晓阳、高希言、常小荣、张洪涛、吕明庄、王玲玲、宣丽华、翟伟、岗卫娟、王昕、董国锋、王芳。

本部分首次发布于 2011 年，本次为第一次修订。

引　言

《循证针灸临床实践指南》是根据针灸临床优势，针对特定临床情况，参照古代文献、名医经验以及现代最佳临床研究证据，结合患者价值观和意愿，系统研制的帮助临床医生和患者做出恰当针灸处理的指导性意见。

《循证针灸临床实践指南》制定的总体思路是：在针灸实践与临床研究的基础上，遵循循证医学的理念与方法，紧紧围绕针灸临床的特色优势，综合专家经验、目前最佳证据以及患者价值观，将国际公认的证据质量评价与推荐方案分级的规范与古代、前人、名老针灸专家临床证据相结合，并将临床研究证据与大范围专家共识相结合，旨在制定出能保障针灸临床疗效和安全性，并具有科学性与实用性的可有效指导针灸临床实践的指导性意见。

在《循证针灸临床实践指南》的制定过程中，各专家组共同参与，还完成了国家标准《针灸临床实践指南制定与评估规范》（以下简称《规范》）的送审稿。《规范》参照了国际上临床实践指南制定的要求和经验，根据中国国情以及针灸的发展状况，对《循证针灸临床实践指南》制定的组织、人员、过程、采用证据质量评价、推荐方案等级划分、专家共识形成方式、制定与更新的内容和时间等都进行了规范。这些规范性要求在《循证针灸临床实践指南》制定中都得到了充分考量与完善。《规范》与《循证针灸临床实践指南》相辅相成，《规范》是《循证针灸临床实践指南》制定的指导，《循证针灸临床实践指南》又是《规范》适用性的验证实例。

《循证针灸临床实践指南》推荐等级主要采用世界卫生组织（WHO）等推荐的 GRADE（Grading of Recommendations Assessment, Development and Evaluation）系统，即推荐分级的评价、制定与评估的系统，其中推荐等级分为强推荐与弱推荐两级。强推荐的方案是估计变化可能性较小，个性化程度低的方案，而弱推荐方案则是估计变化可能性较大，个性化程度高，患者价值观差异大的方案。对于古代文献和名医经验的证据质量评价，目前课题组还在进一步研制中，《循证针灸临床实践指南》仅将古代文献和名医经验作为证据之一附列在现代证据后面，供《循证针灸临床实践指南》使用者参考。

2008 年，在 WHO 西太区的项目资助下，由中国中医科学院牵头、中国针灸学会标准化工作委员会组织完成了针灸治疗带状疱疹、贝尔面瘫、抑郁症、中风后假性球麻痹和偏头痛 5 种病症的指南研制工作。在这 5 种病症的指南研制过程中，课题组初步提出了《循证针灸临床实践指南》的研究方法和建议，建立了《循证针灸临床实践指南》的体例、研究模式与技术路线。2010 年 12 月，《临床病症中医临床实践指南·针灸分册》由中国中医药出版社正式出版发行。

2009 年至 2013 年，在国家中医药管理局立项支持下，中国针灸学会标准化工作委员会又先后分 3 批启动了 15 种病症的指南研制工作。为了保证《循证针灸临床实践指南》高质量地完成，在总课题组的组织下，由四川大学华西医院吴泰相教授在京举办两次 GRADE 方法学培训会议，全国 11 家临床及科研单位的 100 多位学员接受了培训。随后，总课题组又组织了 15 个疾病临床指南制定课题组和 1 个方法学课题组中的 17 位研究人员，赴华西医院循证医学中心接受了为期 3 个月的 Meta 分析和 GRADE 方法学专题培训，受训研究人员系统学习并掌握了 GRADE 系统证据质量评价和推荐意见形成的方法。

本次出版的《循证针灸临床实践指南》共有 20 个部分，包括对 2010 年版 5 部分指南的修订再版和 2013 年完成的 15 部分指南的首次出版。《循证针灸临床实践指南》的适用对象为从事针灸临床与科研的专业人员。

《循证针灸临床实践指南》的证据质量分级和推荐强度等级如下：

◇证据质量分级

证据质量高：A

证据质量中：B

证据质量低：C

证据质量极低：D

◇推荐强度等级

支持使用某项干预措施的强推荐：1

支持使用某项干预措施的弱推荐：2

《循证针灸临床实践指南》的编写，凝聚着全国针灸标准化科研人员和管理人员的辛勤汗水，是参与研制各方集体智慧的结晶，是辨证论治的个体化诊疗模式与循证医学有机结合的创造性探索。《循证针灸临床实践指南》在研制过程中，得到了兰州大学循证医学中心杨克虎教授、陈耀龙博士以及北京大学循证医学中心詹思延教授在方法学上的大力支持和帮助，在此深表感谢。同时，还要感谢国家中医药管理局政策法规与监督司领导的热心指导与大力支持；此外，还要感谢各位专家的通力合作；在《循证针灸临床实践指南》的出版过程中，中国中医药出版社表现出了很高的专业水平，在此一并致谢。

摘　　要

1　治疗原则

针灸治疗中风后假性球麻痹的总原则为辨证治疗。

中风后假性球麻痹以吞咽困难和构音障碍为主要临床表现，针灸治疗中风后假性球麻痹以对症选穴为主，结合循经远端选穴和/或辨证选穴。对症选穴通常选取项部和颈部的穴位。

对于吞咽功能 0～1 级的患者，在使用鼻饲管的同时，建议尽早开始针灸治疗；在吞咽功能达到 2 级或以上时，可以拔除鼻饲管，针灸治疗的同时需配合吞咽功能康复训练，以促进吞咽功能康复。

2　主要推荐意见

推荐意见		推荐级别
中风后各期假性球麻痹患者推荐采用体针疗法		强推荐
中风后各期假性球麻痹患者推荐采用项针疗法		强推荐
中风后各期假性球麻痹患者推荐采用醒脑开窍疗法		强推荐
中风后各期假性球麻痹患者推荐采用头体针结合疗法，尤其适用于中风恢复期、后遗症期以半身不遂、假性球麻痹为主症者		强推荐
中风后各期假性球麻痹患者可采用放血疗法，尤其适用于吞咽功能障碍明显者		弱推荐
中风后各期假性球麻痹患者可采用靳三针疗法		弱推荐
中风后各期假性球麻痹患者可采用任督通调针刺法，尤其适用于吞咽功能障碍明显者		弱推荐
中风后各期假性球麻痹患者，根据具体病情可以酌情选用穴组方案	针对主症近部选穴，含颈部取穴、项部取穴、咽及舌部位取穴	强推荐
	循经远端取穴	弱推荐
	辨证选穴	弱推荐
中风后各期假性球麻痹患者推荐采用针刺结合康复疗法		强推荐

简　介

《循证针灸临床实践指南：中风后假性球麻痹》（以下简称《指南》）简介如下：

1　本《指南》制定的目标

本《指南》制定的目标是制定高质量、体现针灸学科特色的针灸临床实践指南。

2　本《指南》制定的目的

本《指南》制定的目的在于规范中风后假性球麻痹的针灸治疗方案，为临床提供在一般情况下适用于大多数患者的临床实践策略，以提高针灸治疗本病的安全性和有效性。

3　本《指南》的适用人群

本《指南》的适用人群主要为执业中医师和执业助理中医师、医学院校的教师和学生、针灸科研人员。

本《指南》适用的目标环境包括国内各级医院针灸科门诊部或住院部、有针灸专业医师的社区医院、有针灸专业的高等院校、各针灸相关的科研及评价机构。

4　本《指南》适用的疾病范围

本《指南》适用于中风后假性球麻痹患者的针灸治疗，真性球麻痹患者亦可参考本《指南》进行针灸治疗。

概　述

1　定义

1.1　西医

假性球麻痹（pseudobulbar paralysis，PBP）又称中枢性延髓麻痹或上运动神经元性延髓麻痹，多见于脑梗死患者急性期，是指脑桥或脑桥以上部位发生病变，造成延脑内运动神经核失去上位神经支配，而出现以吞咽困难、饮水呛咳、构音障碍为主的一组病症。本《指南》主要介绍中风后假性球麻痹。

1.2　中医

传统中医学没有"假性球麻痹"这一病名，根据西医对假性球麻痹的定义及临床症状等方面的相关描述，中风后假性球麻痹可以归属于中医学"舌喑""喑痱""喑哑""舌蹇"等范畴。

2　发病率

1986～1990年流行病学调查显示，中国脑卒中发病率为（109.7～217）/10万[1]，而脑卒中后有14%（大脑半球）～71%（脑干）的患者伴发假性球麻痹吞咽障碍[2]。英国杂志报道，脑卒中后45%的患者发生吞咽障碍[3]，其中有误吸的中、重度吞咽障碍的发生率高达33%[4]。凡发生在皮质至脑干之间任何部位的脑出血、脑梗死，影响到双侧上运动神经元的功能，都可以引起假性球麻痹。

临床特点

1 病史

中风后假性球麻痹由中风后双侧上运动神经元病损造成，最常见的病因是高血压及动脉硬化性脑血管病，尤其多见于反复发作的双侧脑血管病。既往有单侧脑卒中病史的患者再次发作脑卒中时，假性球麻痹的发生率明显增高。其原因可能为单侧脑卒中时对侧神经细胞功能代偿而不出现症状，双侧受损或再次卒中损害对侧皮质脑干束时，都可出现假性球麻痹。

2 症状及体征

中风后假性球麻痹患者主要临床表现为构音障碍和吞咽障碍。构音障碍主要表现为声音嘶哑、言语不清、同语反复和原有音色改变。吞咽障碍轻者饮水时偶尔或经常呛咳，张口困难，舌不能把食物送至咽部，仰卧位时可以缓慢吞咽；重者完全不能吞咽。神经系统检查示：咽反射存在，无肌萎缩，下颌反射亢进，掌颌反射阳性，叩唇反射阳性，腱反射亢进，常伴有锥体束征阳性等。

3 预防和早期发现

中风后假性球麻痹多见于多次或多处、双侧脑卒中，因此本病的预防关键是防止脑卒中的发生；对于首次发生脑卒中者，要预防复发；对于已经发生假性球麻痹的患者，针灸治疗要及早介入，争取尽早康复。

诊断标准

1 西医诊断标准[5]

1.1 吞咽障碍

轻者饮水时偶尔或经常呛咳，张口困难，舌不能把食物送至咽部，仰卧位时可以缓慢吞咽；重者完全不能吞咽。

1.2 构音障碍

音调拖长缓慢，字句简单。

1.3 神经系统检查

咽反射存在，下颌反射亢进，掌颌反射阳性，叩唇反射阳性，腱反射亢进。

1.4 脑部 CT 或 MRI 检查

脑桥以上两个或多发性病灶。

1.5 其他

常伴有强哭或强笑。

2 中医病/证相关的诊断[6]

2.1 风痰阻络型

声音嘶哑，语言不清或舌暗失语，呛咳频作，吞咽不利，口角流涎，舌体短缩偏斜，苔厚腻，脉弦滑。

2.2 肝阳上亢型

言语不利，舌强语謇，吞咽不利，头胀而痛，烦躁不安，舌歪，舌颤，脉弦数或弦滑。

2.3 肾精亏虚型

声音嘶哑，言语不清或不能言语，吞咽困难，食则呛咳，头晕耳鸣，腰膝酸软，舌体痿软，舌歪，脉弦细或细数。

2.4 瘀血阻窍型

咽喉与腭舌肌瘫痪，吞咽困难，声音嘶哑，口唇紫暗，舌质紫暗或有瘀斑，脉细涩。

3 吞咽功能状态分级[5]

4 级：吞咽运动正常。

3 级：饮水时有呛咳，进食尚好。

2 级：饮水经常呛咳（每次可饮 3 小勺以内，每勺约 2mL），进食缓慢。

1 级：饮水困难（饮 5 勺水有 3 次呛咳），需靠鼻饲流食为主。

0 级：吞咽运动丧失，完全依靠鼻饲流食。

4 言语功能状态分级[5]

4 级：言语流利，音量正常，内容明确，交流能力完全。

3 级：言语较流利，音量小，内容明确，交流能力较全。

2 级：言语不流利，音量弱，内容较明确，交流能力不完全。

1 级：言语断续，听不清，内容不明确，交流能力丧失。

0 级：无言语动作。

5 鉴别诊断[6]

假性球麻痹与真性球麻痹的鉴别：真性球麻痹为下运动神经元性延髓麻痹，有舌肌萎缩，肌纤维颤动，咽反射消失；假性球麻痹为上运动神经元性延髓麻痹，无舌肌萎缩，无肌纤维颤动，咽反射存在，下颌反射亢进。并可根据病史和辅助检查，帮助进行鉴别诊断。

针灸治疗概况

1 现代文献

　　针灸治疗中风后假性球麻痹的总原则为对症治疗。治疗 5～15 天为 1 个疗程，根据每个治疗方案中疗程长短的不同，连续治疗 1～3 个疗程。针灸治疗中风后假性球麻痹以改善吞咽困难和构音障碍为主要目的，一般认为，中风后假性球麻痹针刺干预的时机宜在发病后 20 天内。

　　中风后假性球麻痹以吞咽困难和构音障碍为主要临床表现，现代文献一般根据其临床症状以对症选穴治疗为主，结合循经远端选穴和/或辨证选穴。针对主症近部选穴：通常选取项部和颈部的穴位。根据本病病位在脑，累及舌咽的特点，颈部常用腧穴有廉泉、夹廉泉、人迎、扶突等，项部常用腧穴有风池、风府、哑门、完骨等。病情轻者，可以项部腧穴为主；病情重者，建议颈、项部腧穴同用。循经远端选穴：循行至咽喉部的经脉有足少阴肾经、足阳明胃经、足厥阴肝经、手太阴肺经、阴阳跷脉等，常用的腧穴如列缺、照海、通里、丰隆、三阴交、内关等穴。辨证选穴：根据不同的辨证分型，选取相应的腧穴。如肝阳上亢配太冲，风痰阻络配丰隆，瘀血阻窍配足三里、三阴交，肾精亏虚配太溪、太冲等。总之针灸治疗中风后假性球麻痹要以对症选穴为主。重视对症选穴与辨证选穴相结合，近部选穴与远端选穴相结合。针对中风后假性球麻痹常见并发症选穴治疗也是针灸治疗中风后假性球麻痹的内容之一。中风后假性球麻痹首先要重点治疗主要症状，同时不能忽视并发症的治疗。中风后假性球麻痹是由于双侧上运动神经元损伤所造成的，病因中最常见的是高血压和动脉硬化性脑血管病，尤其是反复发作的双侧脑血管病，因此临床上常见偏侧肢体功能活动障碍、吞咽困难和构音障碍、情感障碍、认知障碍等。中风后假性球麻痹伴有偏瘫的患者在针对主症治疗的同时，可以配伍肩髃、曲池、外关、合谷、后溪、环跳、足三里、阳陵泉、悬钟等；伴有强哭强笑者，配伍百会、印堂、人中等；伴有中枢性尿失禁者，配伍四神聪、百会。在治疗频度上，大多数文献报道每日治疗 1 次，5～15 次为 1 个疗程，疗程间休息 1～2 天。一般连续治疗 1～3 个疗程。目前对针灸治疗中风后假性球麻痹的干预时机尚没有明确结论，但从临床研究文献看，介入治疗最早者为发病 1 日内，并无不良反应。一般认为，中风后假性球麻痹采用针刺干预的时间越早越好，发病 20 天内针刺，其疗效优于 20 天后才进行针灸治疗，但发病 10 天内与 11～20 天内开始治疗相比，疗效差异不明显，此结论还有待进一步临床验证。

2 古代文献

　　共查阅到 32 部关于针灸治疗类似假性球麻痹的古代文献，古代文献记载多以单穴为主，涉及 61 个腧穴共 359 穴次，其中近部选穴 20 个，使用频次为 198 次。近部选穴以督脉、任脉手阳明大肠经、手太阳小肠经等经脉为主，远端选穴以手阳明大肠经、手少阴心经、手少阳三焦经、足少阴肾经等经脉为主，多数文献没有提及辨证配穴、刺灸方法及针灸疗程等内容。

3 名医经验

　　在名医经验的文献记载中，多以腧穴处方的形式出现。文献多出现在名医专著、经验集及教材中，有完整的刺灸方法、疗程等内容，治疗方法主要包括针刺、头针、放血等。

针灸治疗和推荐方案

1 针灸治疗的原则及特点

1.1 治疗总则

针灸治疗中风后假性球麻痹的总原则为对症治疗。

治疗 5～15 天为 1 个疗程，根据每个治疗方案中疗程长短的不同，连续治疗 1～3 个疗程。

针灸治疗中风后假性球麻痹以改善吞咽困难和构音障碍为主要目的，目前对针灸治疗中风后假性球麻痹的干预时机尚没有明确结论，但从临床研究文献看，介入治疗最早者为发病 1 日内[8]，并无不良反应。一般认为，中风后假性球麻痹采用针刺干预的时间越早越好[9]，发病 20 天内针刺，其疗效优于 20 天后才进行针灸治疗，但发病 10 天内与 11～20 天内开始治疗相比，疗效差异不明显[46]，此结论还有待进一步临床验证。

1.2 选穴处方特点

中风后假性球麻痹以吞咽困难和构音障碍为主要临床表现，针灸治疗中风后假性球麻痹建议以对症选穴为主，结合循经远端选穴和/或辨证选穴。

1.2.1 针对主症近部选穴

通常选取项部和颈部的穴位。根据本病病位在脑，累及舌咽的特点，颈部常用腧穴有廉泉、夹廉泉、人迎、扶突等，项部常用腧穴有风池、风府、哑门、完骨等。病情轻者，可以项部腧穴为主；病情重者，建议颈、项部腧穴同用。具体见图 1 至图 3[7]。

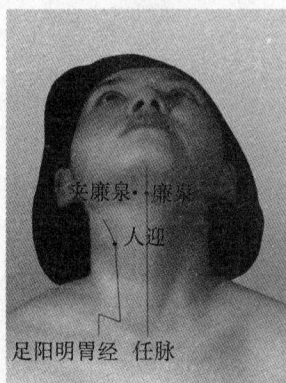

图 1 头颈部经络
腧穴示意图（正面）　　　图 2 头项部经络
腧穴示意图（背面）　　　图 3 头颈部经络
腧穴示意图（右侧位）

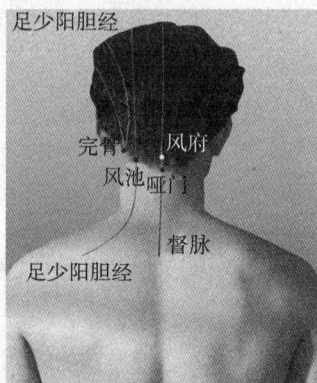

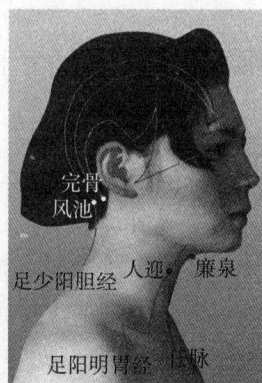

1.2.2 循经远端选穴

循行至咽喉部的经脉有足少阴肾经、足阳明胃经、足厥阴肝经、手太阴肺经、阴阳跷脉等，常用的腧穴如列缺、照海、通里、丰隆、三阴交、内关等穴。

1.2.3 辨证选穴

根据不同的辨证分型[6]，选取相应的腧穴。如肝阳上亢配太冲，风痰阻络配丰隆，瘀血阻窍配足三里、三阴交，肾精亏虚配太溪、太冲等。

针灸治疗中风后假性球麻痹要以对症选穴为主。重视对症选穴与辨证选穴相结合，近部选穴与远端选穴相结合。

1.2.4 针对并发症选穴

中风后假性球麻痹是由于双侧上运动神经元损伤所造成的，病因中最常见的是高血压和动脉硬化性脑血管病，尤其是反复发作的双侧脑血管病，因此临床上常见偏侧肢体功能活动障碍、吞咽困难和构音障碍、情感障碍、认知障碍等。

中风后假性球麻痹首先要重点治疗主要症状，同时不能忽视并发症的治疗。中风后假性球麻痹伴有偏瘫的患者在针对主症治疗的同时，可以配伍肩髃、曲池、外关、合谷、后溪、环跳、足三里、阳陵泉、悬钟等；伴有强哭强笑者，配伍百会、印堂、人中等；伴有中枢性尿失禁者，配伍四神聪、百会。

2 主要结局指标

2.1 有效性评价

根据《中医病证诊断疗效标准·中风诊断疗效评定标准》提及的吞咽言语功能状态评价等疗效评价指标评价的结果表明，针灸治疗中风后假性球麻痹能明显改善患者的吞咽、言语功能[11-13]。

在查阅的所有文献中，均无有关患者依从性的记录，所以不能明确总结出患者对针灸治疗的依从性。但是，一般来讲，患者的依从性主要与不良反应和疗效有关。目前的文献表明，针灸治疗效果显著，且未见明显不良反应。

2.2 卫生经济学评价

根据检索到的文献，目前尚无关于针灸治疗中风后假性球麻痹卫生经济学的分析和描述。

2.3 生活质量评价

在检索到的文献中，尚未有文献对假性球麻痹患者生活质量进行系统评价，但在部分对中风患者生存质量进行评价的文献中，有证据表明，中医综合方法能改善中风患者的生存质量[14]。

2.4 不良反应

在检索到的文献中，绝大多数文献没有明确地对针灸治疗中风后假性球麻痹的不良反应进行观察及报道。有少量临床研究文献报道[9,15]，针刺过程中未见明显的不良反应。有一篇文献报道[16]，针刺过程中未出现晕厥、心律失常等异常情况。

3 注意事项

3.1 操作注意事项

对于吞咽功能0~1级的患者，建议尽早针灸治疗，但不拔除鼻饲管；在吞咽功能达到2级或以上时，可以拔除鼻饲管，针灸治疗时需配合吞咽功能康复训练，以促进吞咽功能康复；对于针感耐受性不强的患者，临床不可给予过强刺激；脑出血行开颅术的患者，头部取穴宜避免在手术区内进行。使用电针治疗时的具体操作注意事项，参照电针操作要求。

关于中风后假性球麻痹构音障碍的针灸治疗，尚需进一步的研究支持。

3.2 禁忌证

在检索到的文献中，未见针灸治疗中风后假性球麻痹禁忌证的明确记录和报道。针灸治疗中风后假性球麻痹的禁忌证和注意事项可以参照针材中的相关内容。对于安装有心脏起搏器的中风后假性球麻痹患者，不宜用电针；对于应用鼻饲管进食的本病患者，在针刺项部时，不宜进针过深。

4 推荐方案

4.1 穴组方案推荐

经过对针灸治疗中风后假性球麻痹文献的学习、分析发现，虽然各处方中的腧穴不尽相同，但某些腧穴常常同时出现在不同的处方中，即常以相对固定的穴组的形式见于各针灸处方中。故本《指南》以穴组方案的形式予以推荐。

4.1.1 针对主症近部选穴

颈部取穴

廉泉、夹廉泉、人迎、扶突位于颈部，与咽喉相邻，能够疏通咽喉部经络气血，有利咽开音之效。属于近部选穴范畴。现代医学认为颈部腧穴能改善颈内动脉供血，促进脑功能的恢复。中风后假性球麻痹患者若出现吞咽障碍或构音障碍者，均可采用本穴。

取穴：廉泉、夹廉泉、人迎、扶突。

针刺操作：人迎，位于喉结尖旁开1.5寸，颈总动脉内侧缘，直刺1~1.5寸，局部有窒息样针感。廉泉，施以合谷刺法，先向舌根方向刺入1.5~1.8寸，再向左右各刺入1.5~1.8寸，以局部得气为宜。夹廉泉，位于廉泉同一水平旁开0.5寸，针尖向舌根方向，进针1.2~1.5寸，局部有酸胀感即可。扶突，向喉头方向斜刺，深约1寸，以针感向喉头放射为佳。以上4穴均在得气后施以平补平泻手法。

电针操作：双侧夹廉泉可以接电针治疗仪，采用疏密波，以病人能耐受为度。

穴位注射操作：在廉泉穴进行穴位注射。令患者仰卧，用5mL注射器抽取药液（临床常用B族维生素），7号长针头注射。针尖朝向舌根方向刺入2寸左右，舌体有针感后推入药液，每穴1mL。

颈部取穴横断面解剖图见图4、图5[7]。

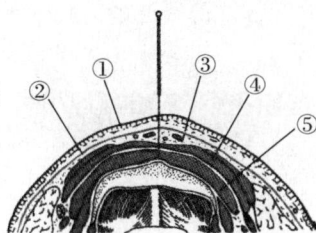

图4 廉泉穴横断面图示
①皮肤；②皮下组织；③针在左、右二腹肌前腹之间通过；④下颌舌骨肌；⑤颏舌骨肌

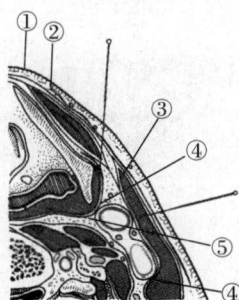

图5 人迎穴横断面图示
①皮肤；②皮下组织和颈阔肌；③颈固有筋膜浅层及胸锁乳突肌；④颈固有筋膜深层；⑤咽缩肌

疗程：每日1次，5次为1个疗程，连续治疗2~3个疗程。

注意事项：①针刺颈项部穴位要特别注意针刺的深度和方向。针刺人迎时，应避开颈总动脉。②严格遵守电针操作的相关注意事项。

『推荐』

> 推荐建议：廉泉、夹廉泉、人迎、扶突主要用于改善患者吞咽功能及构音功能。[GRADE 1C]

解释：本《指南》小组共纳入现代文献3篇、名老中医经验3篇、古代文献2部，经综合分析，形成证据体发现，本方案能明显改善中风后假性球麻痹患者的吞咽功能和语言功能。证据体质量等级经GRADE评价后，因其纳入文献设计质量低、不一致性、不精确性及存在发表偏倚而降低，最终证据体质量等级为低。结合专家共识意见，给予强推荐。

项部取穴

风府、哑门、风池、百劳均位于项部，风府、哑门属于督脉，风池属于胆经，百劳穴为经外奇穴，针刺诸穴具有调节咽喉部气血、发挥利咽开音的作用，是治疗言语不利及吞咽障碍的常用穴，属于近部选穴。研究发现，针刺项部腧穴能改善椎基底动脉供血，促进脑功能恢复。中风后假性球麻痹患者若出现吞咽障碍或构音障碍者，均可选用这些腧穴。

取穴：风府、风池、哑门、百劳。

针刺操作：风府，针尖朝向喉结方向，进针 1 ~ 1.2 寸。风池，针尖稍向内下方，刺入 1 ~ 1.5 寸。哑门，针尖向下颌方向缓慢刺入 0.5 ~ 1 寸。百劳，直刺 1.2 寸。诸穴以局部有酸胀感为宜。

电针操作：双侧风池可以接电针治疗仪，采用疏密波，电流强度以病人能耐受为度。

穴位注射操作：在风池、哑门进行穴位注射。用 5mL 注射器抽取药液（临床常用 B 族维生素），以 7 号长针头针刺，进针得气后每穴注射药液 1mL。

以上 3 种治疗方法，可以单独选用，也可以选择 2 ~ 3 种结合使用。

项部取穴横断面解剖见图 6、图 7[7]。

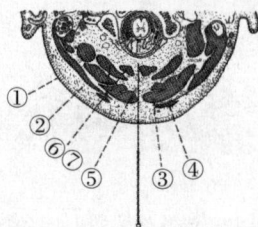

图 6　风府穴横断面解剖图示
①皮肤；②皮下组织；③斜方肌腱；④头半棘肌；⑤项韧带；⑥头后小直肌；⑦头后大直肌

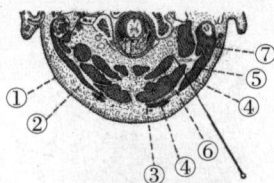

图 7　风池穴横断面解剖图示
①皮肤；②皮下组织；③斜方肌和胸锁乳突肌之间通过；④头夹肌；
⑤头半棘肌；⑥针的内侧为头后大直肌；⑦针的外侧为头上斜肌

疗程：每日 1 次，5 次为 1 个疗程，连续治疗 2 ~ 3 个疗程。

注意事项：①风府、哑门不可向上斜刺过深，以免伤及深部延髓；②严格遵守电针操作的相关注意事项。

『推荐』

推荐建议：风府、风池、哑门、百劳穴主要用于改善患者吞咽功能及构音功能。[GRADE 1C]

解释：本《指南》小组共纳入现代文献 2 篇、名老中医经验 2 篇、古代文献 2 部，经综合分析，形成证据体发现，本方案能明显改善中风后假性球麻痹患者的吞咽功能和构音功能。证据体质量等级经 GRADE 评价后，因其纳入文献设计质量低、不一致性、不精确性及存在发表偏倚而降低，最终证据体质量等级为低。结合专家共识意见，给予强推荐。

咽、舌部位取穴

刺激咽后壁能恢复和重建吞咽反射弧，对吞咽功能障碍有改善作用。金津、玉液位于舌下，能调节舌肌功能，是针灸治疗言语不利的常用穴位，均属于局部选穴范畴。以上三穴多采用点刺放血法治疗，对无出血倾向的中风后假性球麻痹患者，均可采用此疗法。

取穴：咽后壁、金津、玉液。

针刺操作：咽后壁，令患者张口，用压舌板将舌体向后下方推压，以长度75～100mm的芒针点刺悬雍垂两侧之咽后壁，每侧3～5针，少量出血，不留针。金津、玉液，让患者自然将舌伸出口外（如舌不能伸出者，医者可用纱布牵拉、固定舌体于口外），常规消毒二穴，用粗毫针或三棱针点刺，使少量出血，不留针。

疗程：每日1次，10次为1个疗程，连续治疗2个疗程。

注意事项：①点刺后令患者保持低头位，避免血液回流气管引发呼吸道堵塞；②有出血倾向患者慎用此法。

『推荐』

> 推荐建议：咽后壁点刺放血对中风后假性球麻痹吞咽障碍有明显改善作用。金津、玉液点刺放血对构音障碍有明显改善作用。可根据患者是否具有吞咽障碍、构音障碍表现单独选用或结合选用。［GRADE 1B］

解释：本《指南》小组共纳入现代文献3篇、名老中医经验2篇，经综合分析，形成证据体发现，本方案能明显改善中风后假性球麻痹患者的吞咽功能和语言功能。证据体质量等级经GRADE评价后，因其纳入文献设计质量低、不一致性、不精确性及存在发表偏倚而降低，最终证据体质量等级为中等。结合专家共识意见，给予强推荐。

4.1.2　循经远端取穴

根据"经络所过，主治所及"的原则，针灸治疗中风后假性球麻痹可以配合循经远端选取腧穴进行针灸治疗。根据文献报道，常用的4组对穴如下。治疗时可选择其中1～2组作为配穴使用。

取穴：列缺与照海，通里与内关，丰隆与三阴交，合谷与太冲。

针刺操作：以上腧穴常规针刺，施以平补平泻手法。

电针操作：丰隆与三阴交、合谷与太冲可以接电针治疗仪，采用疏密波，以病人能耐受为度。

疗程：每日1次，10次为1个疗程，连续治疗2个疗程。

注意事项：①同常规针刺的注意事项；②严格遵守电针操作的相关注意事项。

『推荐』

> 推荐建议：循经远端取穴是针灸治疗中风后假性球麻痹腧穴处方的重要组成部分，一般是在针对主症局部选穴的基础上，作为配穴选用，可以增强疗效。通常选择1～2组。［GRADE 2B］

解释：本《指南》小组共纳入现代文献4篇，经综合分析，形成证据体发现，循经远端取穴能帮助改善中风后假性球麻痹患者的吞咽功能和语言功能。证据体质量等级经GRADE评价后，因其纳入文献设计质量低、不一致性、不精确性及存在发表偏倚而降低，最终证据体质量等级为中等。结合专家共识意见，给予弱推荐。

4.1.3　辨证选穴

辨证选穴是针灸选穴处方的依据之一，体现了治病求本的中医诊治思维特点。针灸治疗中风后假性球麻痹也可以配合辨证取穴进行针灸治疗。根据文献报道，常用的辨证选穴如下，治疗时可根据辨证结果相应地选择配穴。

取穴：肝阳上亢加太冲、太溪，风痰阻络配丰隆、中脘，瘀血阻窍配足三里、三阴交，肾精亏虚配太溪、肾俞。

针刺操作：根据"虚则补之，实则泻之"的原则，太冲、丰隆、三阴交施提插捻转泻法，足三里、太溪、肾俞施提插捻转补法。

电针操作：根据辨证选用一组穴位，接通电针治疗仪，采用疏密波，以病人能耐受为度。

疗程：每日1次，10次为1个疗程，连续治疗2个疗程。

注意事项：①对于虚证患者施予电针治疗时，电流强度不宜过大；②严格遵守电针操作的相关注意事项。

『推荐』

> 推荐建议：辨证选穴是针灸治疗中风后假性球麻痹腧穴处方的重要组成部分，一般是在针对主症局部选穴的基础上，作为配穴选用，对于治病求本、巩固临床疗效有重要意义。［GRADE 2D］

解释：本《指南》小组共纳入现代文献3篇，经综合分析，形成证据体发现，辨证选穴能帮助改善中风后假性球麻痹患者的吞咽功能和语言功能。证据体质量等级经GRADE评价后，因其纳入文献设计质量低、不一致性、不精确性及存在发表偏倚而降低，最终证据体质量等级为极低。结合专家共识意见，给予弱推荐。

4.2 处方方案推荐

根据患者情况，可以选取上述推荐的一种或两种以上的穴组方案，构成治疗中风后假性球麻痹的针灸处方。

4.2.1 体针疗法

体针疗法是针灸治疗中风后假性球麻痹最常见的治疗方法，选穴以对局部症选穴为主，根据需要可以适当辨证选穴配伍治疗，操作上以毫针刺法为主，可以配合电针法等其他治疗方法。

取穴：风府、百劳、人迎、廉泉、夹廉泉。

针刺操作：具体针刺方法可见本章节4.1.1中"颈部取穴"与"项部取穴"的内容。

电针操作：针刺得气后，夹廉泉接通电针治疗仪，采用疏密波，以患者能耐受为度。

疗程：每日治疗1次，连续治疗15次为1个疗程，连续治疗1~2个疗程。

注意事项：①高血压病患者，针刺人迎时针感不宜过强；②严格遵守电针操作的相关注意事项。

『推荐』

> 推荐建议：本方案适用于中风各期的假性球麻痹患者。［GRADE 1B］

解释：本《指南》小组共纳入相关文献5篇，经综合分析，形成证据体发现，本方案能明显改善中风后假性球麻痹患者的吞咽功能和语言功能。证据体质量等级经GRADE评价后，因其纳入文献设计质量低、不一致性、不精确性及存在发表偏倚而降低，最终证据体质量等级为中等。结合专家共识意见，给予强推荐。

4.2.2 项针疗法

项针疗法是黑龙江中医药大学附属第一医院高维滨教授等创立的一种特殊针灸疗法，用于治疗假性球麻痹疗效显著。自1996年至今已有多年的临床应用经验，目前在国内东北地区应用较广，其他部分地区也有应用。

取穴：风池、翳明、治呛（甲状软骨上切迹上缘与舌骨下缘之间，直刺1寸以内）、供血（风池穴直下1.5寸，向内侧直刺1寸）、吞咽（喉结与舌骨体中点，旁开0.5寸，向内侧稍斜刺0.3寸）、发音（甲状软骨与环状软骨的中点，旁开0.2寸，直刺0.3寸）、治反流（发音穴外0.5寸，向内侧斜刺0.3寸）、廉泉、外金津、玉液。

针刺操作：风池、翳明、供血，针尖稍向内下方，刺入1~1.5寸。廉泉、外金津、玉液，向舌根刺入 1.2～1.5 寸。治呛、吞咽，直刺 0.3 寸。发音、治反流穴，直刺 0.2 寸。

疗程：每日上、下午各治疗 1 次。5 天为 1 个疗程，疗程间休息 1 天，连续治疗 2～3 个疗程。

注意事项：①同常规针刺注意事项；②严格遵守电针操作的相关注意事项。

『推荐』

推荐建议：本方案适用于中风各期的假性球麻痹患者。[GRADE 1B]

解释：本《指南》小组共纳入相关文献 3 篇，经综合分析，形成证据体发现，项针疗法能明显改善中风后假性球麻痹患者的吞咽功能和语言功能。证据体质量等级经 GRADE 评价后，因其纳入文献设计质量低、不一致性、不精确性及存在发表偏倚而降低，最终证据体质量等级为低。结合专家共识意见，给予强推荐。

4.2.3 醒脑开窍法

此疗法为天津中医药大学附属第一医院石学敏院士于 1972 年开创的，经过 30 多年的临床反复实践应用，证实有较好的临床疗效。目前国内除天津地区外，许多省、市、县级医院都有应用。

取穴：风池、翳风或完骨、三阴交、内关、水沟。

针刺操作：风池、翳风或完骨，均针向结喉，震颤徐入 2.5 寸，小幅度、高频率捻转 1 分钟，以咽喉部麻胀感为宜。三阴交，直刺 1～1.5 寸，行提插补法 1 分钟。水沟，行雀啄刺，使眼球湿润或流泪为度。内关，行提插捻转泻法 1 分钟。

疗程：首次治疗先刺水沟、内关，以后可 2～3 天针刺 1 次；风池、翳风或完骨、三阴交每日 1 次。10 次为 1 个疗程，疗程间休息 2 天，连续治疗 2 个疗程。

注意事项：醒脑开窍法针刺过程中要求出现较强的针感，故应注意避免晕针。体质虚弱患者慎用。

『推荐』

推荐建议：本方案适用于中风各期假性球麻痹患者。[GRADE 1C]

解释：本《指南》小组共纳入相关文献 3 篇，经综合分析，形成证据体发现，醒脑开窍法能明显改善中风后假性球麻痹患者的吞咽功能和语言功能。证据体质量等级经 GRADE 评价后，因其纳入文献设计质量低、不一致性、不精确性及存在发表偏倚而降低，最终证据体质量等级为低。结合专家共识意见，给予强推荐。

4.2.4 头体针结合疗法

此疗法是头针与体针结合，兼具头、体针两种疗法的综合疗效，临床报道疗效较好。

头针取穴：顶中线、顶颞前斜线、顶颞后斜线、顶旁 1 线、顶旁 2 线。

体针取穴：风池、翳风、廉泉、金津、玉液。

头针操作：与头皮呈 15°角斜刺至帽状腱膜下，进针 1～1.5 寸，采用提插手法，进针时幅度小，行针时提插幅度要大。每穴行针约 30 秒，可两针同时操作。边行针边嘱患者尽量活动相应患肢，得气后留针，并连接电针治疗仪，选择断续波，低频，以患者能耐受为度，留针 30 分钟。每日 2 次，上午针患侧，下午针健侧。

体针操作：取风池、翳风、廉泉、金津、玉液。翳风，针尖对准喉结方向进针 2.5 寸。针刺得气后，采用平补平泻手法约 30 秒，留针 30 分钟。

疗程：采用相同的腧穴及操作，上、下午各治疗 1 次。15 天为 1 个疗程，疗程间休息 2 天。共治疗 2 个疗程。

注意事项：脑出血开颅术后患者慎用本法。

『推荐』

> 本方案适用于中风恢复期、后遗症期以半身不遂、假性球麻痹为主症者。[GRADE 1C]

解释：本《指南》小组共纳入相关文献 3 篇，经综合分析，形成证据体发现，头体针结合疗法能明显改善中风后假性球麻痹患者的吞咽功能和语言功能。证据体质量等级经 GRADE 评价后，因其纳入文献设计质量低、不一致性、不精确性及存在发表偏倚而降低，最终证据体质量等级为低。结合专家共识意见，给予强推荐。

4.2.5　放血疗法

此疗法是针灸治疗中风后假性球麻痹的常用方法之一，临床报道疗效较好。在咽后壁点刺放血，其作用与现代医学的咽部冷刺激等吞咽训练有异曲同工的作用，能有效地强化吞咽反射。本疗法适用于中风后假性球麻痹患者。

取穴：咽后壁、翳风、内关。

针刺操作：令患者张口，用压舌板将舌体向后下方推压，以长度 75～100mm 的芒针点刺悬雍垂两侧之咽后壁，每侧 3～5 点，使少量出血，不留针。翳风，向咽部斜刺，进针 2 寸，使麻胀感传至咽部。内关，向肘部斜刺，进针 1.5 寸，使麻胀感传至肘部，留针 20 分钟。

疗程：每日 1 次，10 次为 1 个疗程，疗程间休息 2 日，连续治疗 2 个疗程。

注意事项：有出血倾向患者慎用。

『推荐』

> 推荐建议：本方案适用于中风各期的假性球麻痹患者，尤其适用于吞咽功能障碍明显者。[GRADE 2D]

解释：本《指南》小组共纳入相关文献 3 篇，经综合分析，形成证据体发现，本疗法能明显改善中风后假性球麻痹患者的吞咽功能。证据体质量等级经 GRADE 评价后，因其纳入文献设计质量低、不一致性、不精确性及存在发表偏倚而降低，最终证据体质量等级为极低。结合专家共识意见，给予强推荐。

4.2.6　靳三针疗法

靳三针疗法是靳瑞教授在 40 余年临床实践的基础上，集历代针灸名家临床经验之精华，经反复、系统临床和实验研究总结创造出来的一种针灸流派。其中有适用于中风后假性球麻痹患者的组穴，临床报道疗效较好。

主穴：脑三针（脑户、双侧脑空）和舌三针（上廉泉、上廉泉左右旁开各 1 寸）。

配穴：肝阳暴亢型配足临泣、太冲；风痰阻络型配风市、丰隆；痰热腑实型配曲池、丰隆；气虚血瘀型配足三里、三阴交；阴虚风动型配复溜、太溪。

针刺操作：所有穴位均按常规操作，针刺得气后，行平补平泻手法，配合电针治疗，选疏密波，频率为 2～100Hz。

疗程：每日 1 次，20 次为 1 个疗程，共治疗 1 个疗程。

注意事项：脑出血开颅术后患者慎用脑三针。

『推荐』

> 推荐建议：本方案适用于中风各期的假性球麻痹患者。[CRADE 2D]

解释：本《指南》小组共纳入相关文献 3 篇，经综合分析，形成证据体发现，靳三针疗法能改善中风后假性球麻痹患者的吞咽功能和语言功能。证据体质量等级经 GRADE 评价后，因其纳入文献设计质量低、不一致性、不精确性及存在发表偏倚而降低，最终证据体质量等级为极低。结合专家共识意见，给予弱推荐。

4.2.7　任督通调针刺法

此法是根据任督二脉在循行中与脑和咽喉有密切关系的特点，在此二脉上选取腧穴为主治疗中风后假性球麻痹的一种针刺方法。文献报道显示，能有效改善中风后假性球麻痹患者的吞咽障碍症状，而对患者构音障碍的疗治疗作用，尚待进一步临床验证。

取穴：天突、廉泉、百会、脑户、哑门。

针刺操作：穴位常规消毒。天突，仰靠坐位，取长度40mm的毫针，先直刺0.2寸，当针尖超过胸骨柄内缘后，即向下沿胸骨柄后缘、气管前缘缓慢向下刺入0.5～1寸，然后左手握住针柄缓慢捻转，待患者有闷胀感后慢慢捻转出针。廉泉，取坐位，用长度40mm的毫针，向舌根方向针刺，进针1～1.2寸，以轻手法提插3～5次，得气后将针尖提至皮下，再向咽部方向刺入0.5～0.8寸，以舌根、咽部有酸、痛、胀为佳。百会，取坐位，用长度25mm的毫针，平刺0.5～1寸，捻转2～3次，频率200次/分钟。脑户，取坐位，用长度25mm的毫针，平刺0.5～1寸，捻转2～3次，频率90～120次/分钟。诸穴行针得气后，留针30分钟，其中，廉泉留针期间，每10分钟行平补平泻手法1次。哑门，取坐位，使头微前倾，项肌放松，用长度40mm的毫针，针尖向下颌方向，进针0.5～1寸，施予捻转泻法，频率90～120次/分钟，1分钟后出针。

疗程：每日1次，每周连续治疗6次，休息1天。4周为1个疗程，共治疗1个疗程。

注意事项：①天突穴留针时嘱患者少做吞咽动作；针刺不可过深，以防刺中气管软骨。②哑门不可向上斜刺过深，以免伤及深部延髓。

『推荐』

> 推荐建议：本方案适用于中风各期的假性球麻痹吞咽障碍患者，尤其适用于吞咽功能障碍明显者。[GRADE 2D]

解释：本《指南》小组共纳入相关文献2篇，经综合分析，形成证据体发现，本疗法能改善中风后假性球麻痹患者的吞咽功能。证据体质量等级经GRADE评价后，因其纳入文献设计质量低、不一致性、不精确性及存在发表偏倚而降低，最终证据体质量等级为极低。结合专家共识意见，给予弱推荐。

5　康复与中药治疗

建议参照相关诊疗常规进行，或咨询相关专业科室人员配合共同执行。

参考文献

[1] 王维治. 神经病学 [M]. 北京：人民卫生出版社，2006.

[2] 梁玉宏，张小琳. 卒中急性期的并发症及处理 [J]. 国外医学·脑血管疾病分册，1996，4（1）：39.

[3] Caroline Gordon, Richard Langton hewer, Derick T Wade. Dysphagia in Acute Stroke [J]. British Medical Journal, 1987, 295 (15)：411.

[4] D. G. Smithard, P. A. ONeil, C. Pard, et al, Complications and outcome after acute stroke：Does dysphagia matter [J]. Stroke, 1996, 27 (7)：1200.

[5] 高维滨. 神经病针灸新疗法 [M]. 北京：人民卫生出版社，2002.

[6] 王玉来. 中西医临床神经病学 [M]. 北京：中国中医药出版社，1998.

[7] 严振国. 全身经穴应用解剖图谱 [M]. 上海：上海中医药大学出版社，1997.

[8] 彭华荣. 针刺背俞穴为主治疗假性球麻痹吞咽障碍 40 例 [J]. 辽宁中医学院学报，2005，7（5）：499.

[9] 宋文翔，张春燕. 吞咽复系列穴组针灸治疗脑卒中后吞咽障碍 58 例 [J]. 四川中医，2005，23（7）：107－108.

[10] 孙轩翔，范刚启，戴秀珍. 脑梗死吞咽障碍针刺治疗方案的初步优选 [J]. 中国针灸，2011，31（10）：879－882.

[11] 张志萍，孟进军，吴清明，等. 祛风化痰针刺法治疗假性球麻痹 55 例临床疗效观察 [J]，湖南中医药导报，2003，9（4）：45－47.

[12] 杨国荣. 头体针结合治疗假性延髓麻痹的临床观察 [J]. 上海针灸杂志，2005，24（12）：10－11.

[13] 庞勇，陈尚杰，周开斌，等. 针刺风府穴治疗假性球麻痹 30 例 [J]. 中医杂志，2001，15（11）：817－818.

[14] 刘志顺，王丽平，杨光，等. "调理髓海、通阳柔筋" 针刺法对中风偏瘫患者生存质量及生活自理能力的影响 [J]. 中医杂志，2008，49（2）：138－141.

[15] 刘军，刘志顺，黄石玺，等. 针刺治疗假性球麻痹吞咽障碍临床观察. 中国针灸，1996，16（10）：18.

[16] 高维滨，高金立，王鹏. 项针治疗假性延髓麻痹的临床研究 [J]. 上海针灸杂志，2000，19（6）：14－15.

[17] 刘志顺，刘保延，叶永铭，等. 针刺治疗中风慢性期中重度吞咽障碍临床研究 [J]. 中国针灸，2002，22（5）：291－294.

[18] 沈王明. 扶突穴为主治疗脑卒中假性球麻痹 [J]. 针灸临床杂志，2008，24（3）：17－18.

[19] 石学敏. 石学敏针灸全集 [M]. 北京：科学出版社，2006.

[20] 高维滨. 神经病针灸新疗法 [M]. 北京：人民卫生出版社，2002.

[21] 吕少杰. 神经疾病针灸疗法 [M]. 北京：人民卫生出版社，1999.

[22] 靳宇，李静，马涛. 咽后壁点刺为主治疗假性延髓麻痹 79 例 [J]. 中国针灸，1999（4）：238.

[23] 张惠利. 针刺假性延髓麻痹 102 例临床观察 [J]. 湖北中医药学报，1999，14（2）：32－33.

[24] 石学敏. 针灸治疗学. 第 6 版 [M]. 上海：上海科学技术出版社；1998.

[25] 陈兴华，赖新生，陈治忠. 针刺治疗中风后假性延髓麻痹疗效观察 [J]. 中国针灸，2005，25

（3）：161－162.

［26］钟叙春，刘向红，张梅芳．项针结合腹针治疗脑卒中后假性球麻痹46例［J］．中医杂志，2007，48（1）：55－56.

［27］陈兴华，靳瑞．靳三针治疗中风性假性球麻痹64例疗效观察［J］．新中医，2006，（38）7：65－66.

［28］陈兴华，靳瑞．针刺对中风假性球麻痹患者血液黏稠度的影响［J］．上海针灸杂志，2005，24（2）：7－8.

［29］陈兴华，靳瑞．针刺对中风性假性球麻痹患者血浆内皮素及一氧化氮的影响［J］．针刺研究，2005，30（3），171－174.

［30］张志萍，孟进军，吴清明，等．祛风化痰针刺法治疗假性球麻痹55例临床疗效观察［J］．湖南中医药导报，2003，9（4）：45－47.

［31］刘志顺，黄漫，叶永铭，等．针刺治疗假性球麻痹吞咽障碍临床研究［J］．新中医，1998，30（3）：24－25.

［32］吴清明，冯国湘，刘未艾，等．祛风化痰针刺法治疗风痰型假性球麻痹120例［J］．中国针灸，2005，5（9）：603－606.

［33］冯国湘，刘未艾，曾碧枚．祛风化痰针法对风痰型假性球麻痹患者TCD的影响［J］．上海针灸杂志，2005，9，24（9）：8－10.

［34］刘丽莉，胡淑琴，聂卉，等．项针治疗假性延髓麻痹的SEP变化的动态观察［J］．中国中医药科技，1997，4（2）：75－76.

［35］罗平，张淑忆．项针配合康复训练治疗假性延髓麻痹82例［J］．中国民间疗法，2006，14（5）：50－52，19.

［36］马振河，赵玉成．醒脑开窍针刺法治疗假性球麻痹30例［J］．山东中医杂志，2006，25（6）：397.

［37］曾学清，滕东时，杨涛，等．针刺配合康复训练治疗脑梗塞后构音障碍30例［J］．针灸临床杂志，2005，21（10）：9－10.

［38］郭新民，王宝亮，郭会军．中药配合针灸治疗中风假性球麻痹临床观察［J］．中国医药学报，1997，12（6）：28－29.

［39］刘书鹏，刘华．头针体针治疗脑卒中后假性球麻痹30例［J］．中国民间疗法，2006，14（5）：17－18.

［40］孙华，包飞，王道海，等．头针配合体针治疗中风假性球麻痹疗效观察［J］．中国康复理论与实践，2006，12（7）：599－600.

［41］秦润笋，赵子龙．针刺配合康复训练治疗假性延髓性麻痹30例观察［J］．中国实用神经疾病杂志，2006，9（5）：63－64.

［42］陈晓军，陈利芳，王樟连，等．靳三针治疗中风性假性球麻痹的临床研究［J］．江苏中医药，2010，42（11）62－63.

［43］陈立早，张泓．舌三针联合背俞穴埋线治疗中风后假性球麻痹吞咽困难临床观察［J］．中医药导报，2010，16（7）：72－73.

［44］李飞，程红亮，陈幸生．舌三针为主配合舌肌训练治疗假性球麻痹疗效观察［J］．中医药临床杂志，2012，24（10）：931－932.

［45］苏毅，李佩芳．任督通调针刺法治疗卒中后假性球麻痹吞咽障碍临床研究［J］．中医药临床杂志，2011，23（7）：585－587.

［46］彭长林．任督通调法治疗卒中后假性延髓麻痹疗效观察［J］．中国针灸，2010，30（7）：551－553.

附　　录

1　本《指南》专家组成员和编写组成员

专家组成员

姓名	性别	职称	工作单位	课题中的分工
刘仁权	男	教授	北京中医药大学	文献质量评价和数据的统计分析
谢雁鸣	女	主任医师	中国中医科学院临床基础医学研究所	文献质量评价
高树中	男	教授	山东中医药大学	文献检索方案的制订和临床治疗方案的推荐
吴中朝	男	教授	中国中医科学院针灸医院	文献检索方案的制订和临床治疗方案的推荐
杨　骏	男	教授	安徽中医学院附属医院	文献检索方案的制订和临床治疗方案的推荐
杜元灏	男	教授	天津中医药大学附属医院	文献检索方案的制订和临床治疗方案的推荐

编写组成员

	姓名	性别	学历/职称	工作单位	课题中的分工
组长	赵吉平	女	硕士/教授、主任医师	北京中医药大学东直门医院	草案的起草、组织专家、征求专家意见
秘书	王　军	男	博士/副主任医师	北京中医药大学东直门医院	安排小组会议、征求专家意见、文献检索及数据提取
组员	李　俊	男	博士	解放军463医院	文献检索及整理、提取数据
	白　鹏	男	博士	北京中医药大学东直门医院	文献检索及整理、提取数据
	王　朋	女	硕士	北京中医药大学东直门医院	文献检索及整理、提取数据
	王　鹏	男	硕士	首都医科大学附属北京中医医院	文献检索及整理、提取数据
	郭盛楠	女	博士研究生	北京中医药大学东直门医院	文献检索及整理、提取数据
	陈　晟	男	博士研究生	北京中医药大学东直门医院	文献检索及整理、提取数据
	赵　宏	女	主任医师	中国中医科学院广安门医院	提供证据、推荐等级论证以及文献检索方法学支持
	武晓冬	女	助理研究员	中国中医科学院针灸研究所	提供证据、推荐等级论证以及文献检索方法学支持
	訾明杰	女	实习研究员	中国中医科学院针灸研究所	提供证据、推荐等级论证以及文献检索方法学支持
	郭　旭	男	硕士	中国中医科学院针灸研究所	提供证据、推荐等级论证以及文献检索方法学支

2　临床问题

　　基于适用人群、干预措施、对照、结局和卫生经济学等方面的考虑，由《指南》编写委员会提出本《指南》要解决的临床问题，以医、患问卷调查的形式，进一步对临床问题进行筛选，《指南》制定小组以 PICO 原则产生临床问题，按照四要素进行分解：即研究对象或研究问题（population/problem）、干预措施（intervention）、对照措施（comparator）和结局（outcome）。最终经编写委员会讨论，确定临床关键问题如下：

PICO 项目	PICO 结果
研究对象	中风后假性球麻痹
干预措施	各针灸疗法
对照措施	安慰针、阳性药物、不同针灸疗法
结局指标	见"疗效评价指标分级"

假性球麻痹定义和诊断。

假性球麻痹的病因病机和辨证分型。

假性球麻痹的流行病学和对患者生活的影响。

针灸的最佳干预时机。

针灸治疗方法有哪些？

与其他疗法相比，针灸疗法的优势是什么？

针灸具体操作方法、刺激量、疗程和治疗频次。

针灸具体操作的注意事项。

针灸治疗是否存在不良反应。

是否有助于提高患者的依从性？

是否有助于提高卫生经济学评价？

提供编写《指南》的文献证据级别及推荐等级。

3 疗效评价指标的分级

	指标	采用标准	出现频次	指标等级	备注
临床症状指标	临床症状体征	史玉泉. 实用神经病学［M］. 上海：上海科学技术出版社，1994.	5	7	
	临床症状积分——石氏评分	蒋戈利，石学敏，张存生，等. 醒脑开窍法针刺治疗假性延髓麻痹的临床及实验研究［J］. 天津医药，1992，(3)：168－171.	3	8	
	临床症状积分——洼田饮水实验积分	大西幸子，孙启良. 脑卒中患者摄食－吞咽障碍的评价与训练［J］. 中国康复医学杂志，1997，12 (3)：141－143. 一口量采用20mL可饮用水，评价方法如下：①1次喝完，无呛咳（根据计时又分为：a.5秒之内喝完；b.5秒以上喝完）；②2次以上喝完，无呛咳；③1次喝完，有呛咳；④2次以上喝完，有呛咳；⑤呛咳多次发生，不能将水喝完	1	7	
	中医辨证	国家中医药管理局. 中医病证诊断疗效标准. 南京：南京大学出版社，1994：202.	5	8	
理化指标	颅脑CT或MRI		2	5	
	静脉血血清PGF2α值	采用酶联法测试要求进行测定。PGF2α和PGE2试剂盒由上海森雄科技实业有限公司提供。检测由河北医科大学中心实验室完成	3	5	
	静脉血血清PGE2值	采用酶联法测试要求进行测定。PGF2α和PGE2试剂盒由上海森雄科技实业有限公司提供。检测由河北医科大学中心实验室完成	2	5	
	血浆AVP值	采用放免法测试，由河北医科大学中心实验室完成	1	5	

4 检索范围、检索策略及结果

4.1 检索范围

CNKI 中文数据库，MEDLINE、pubmed、Cochrane 英文数据库，《中华医典》。

4.2 检索策略

4.2.1 现代文献检索策略

（"假性球麻痹 OR 延髓麻痹"）AND（"病因学 OR 影响因素 OR 发病原因 OR 诱因"）

（"假性球麻痹 OR 延髓麻痹"）AND（"针灸 OR 针刺 OR 毫针 OR 灸 OR 电针 OR 耳针 OR 耳穴贴压 OR 水针 OR 皮肤针 OR 皮内针 OR 梅花针 OR 头针 OR 手足针 OR 腕踝针 OR 面针 OR 眼针 OR 温针 OR 刺血疗法 OR 放血疗法 OR 三棱针疗法 OR 蜂针 OR 火针疗法 OR 激光针刺 OR 激光穴位照射 OR 舌针 OR 穴位疗法 OR 穴位按压 OR 点穴 OR 敷脐 OR 拔罐 OR 走罐 OR 闪罐 OR 针药并用"）

（"假性球麻痹 OR 延髓麻痹"）AND（"选穴 OR 取穴 OR 配穴 OR 处方，针灸 OR 针灸处方"）

（"假性球麻痹 OR 延髓麻痹"）AND（"针灸 OR 针刺 OR 毫针 OR 灸 OR 电针 OR 耳针 OR 耳穴贴压 OR 水针 OR 皮肤针 OR 皮内针 OR 梅花针 OR 头针 OR 手足针 OR 腕踝针 OR 面针 OR 眼针 OR 温针 OR 刺血疗法 OR 放血疗法 OR 三棱针疗法 OR 蜂针 OR 火针疗法 OR 激光针刺 OR 激光穴位照射 OR 舌针 OR 穴位疗法 OR 穴位按压 OR 点穴 OR 敷脐 OR 拔罐 OR 走罐 OR 闪罐 OR 针药并用"）AND（"时间因素 OR 时间治疗学 OR 时间医学 OR 择时 OR 子午流注"）

4.2.2 英文文献检索策略

（"Pseudobulbar paralysis OR Supranuclear paralysis"）AND（Etiology OR Causes OR Causality OR "Epidemiologic Factors"）

（"Pseudobulbar paralysis OR Supranuclear paralysis"）AND（Acupuncture OR Acupuncture Therapy OR Needling OR Moxibustion OR Electroacupuncture OR Auriculotherapy OR Hydro－acupuncture OR "Plum－boossom Needle therapy" OR "Intradermal needle therapy" OR "Needle warming therapy" OR "Bloodletting therapy" OR "Three－edged needle therapy" OR Bee－needles OR "Fire－needle therapy" OR Laser OR "Acupoint therapy" OR Acupressure OR "Acupoint sticking therapy" OR "Auricular point sticking" OR Cupping）

（"Pseudobulbar paralysis OR Supranuclear paralysis"）AND（"Point selection" OR "Acupoint selection" OR "Point combination" OR "Acupoint combination" OR "Acupuncture－moxibustion prescription" OR "Acupuncture prescription" OR "Prescription，Acupuncture－moxibustion"）

（"Pseudobulbar paralysis OR Supranuclear paralysis"）AND（Acupuncture OR Needling OR moxibustion OR Electroacupuncture OR Auriculotherapy OR Hydro－acupuncture，OR "Plum－boossom Needle therapy" OR "Intradermal needle therapy" OR "Needle warming therapy" OR "Bloodletting therapy" OR "Three－edged needle therapy" OR Bee－needles OR "Fire－needle therapy" OR Laser OR "Acupoint therapy" OR Acupressure OR "Acupoint sticking therapy" OR "Auricular point sticking" OR Cupping）AND（Time OR "Time factor" OR Chronotherapeuties OR Chronomedicine OR "midnight－noon ebb－flow" OR "Zi Wu Liu Zhu" OR Ziwuliuzhu）

4.2.3 古代文献检索策略

以《中华医典》为搜索工具，以"喑痱/瘖痱/舌缓/喑不能言/舌根紧缩/舌下急/舌蹇/中风不语/喉痹/下食难/（饮）食不下"为关键词，查找古代文献中与假性球麻痹有关的文献记录，并查找原文进行核对。共查询古代医籍32本。分别是：《针灸甲乙经》《备急千金要方》《千金翼方》《医心方》《西方子明堂灸经》《外台秘要》《圣济总录》《太平圣惠方》《幼幼新书》《黄帝明堂灸经》《针灸神书》《针灸资生经》《针经指南》《针经节要》《扁鹊神应针灸玉龙经》《普济方》《针灸聚英》《针灸心法要诀》《针灸大全》《针灸大成》《类经图翼》《古今医统大全》《医学纲目》《卫生宝鉴》

《证治准绳》《重楼玉钥》《凌门传授铜人指穴》《针灸集成》《针灸易学》《针灸逢源》《经络全书》《金针秘传》。

4.2.4 专著文献检索策略

对北京中医药大学图书馆所藏记录中医专家经验的书籍进行查阅，共查询到与针灸治疗假性球麻痹有关的专著4册，分别是：《石学敏针灸全集》《神经病针灸新疗法》《神经疾病针灸疗法》《头皮针治疗学》。

4.3 检索结果

4.3.1 古代文献证据

类似中风后假性球麻痹古代文献见下表。

类似中风后假性球麻痹古代文献

著作	朝代	作者	著作	朝代	作者
1.《针灸甲乙经》	晋	皇甫谧	17.《针灸聚英》	明	高武
2.《备急千金要方》	唐	孙思邈	18.《针灸心法要诀》	明	吴谦，等
3.《千金翼方》	唐	孙思邈	19.《针灸大全》	明	徐凤
4.《医心方》	唐	丹波康赖	20.《针灸大成》	明	杨继洲
5.《西方子明堂灸经》	唐	西方子	21.《类经图翼》	明	张景岳
6.《外台秘要》	唐	王焘	22.《古今医统大全》	明	徐春甫
7.《圣济总录》	宋	赵佶	23.《医学纲目》	明	楼英
8.《太平圣惠方》	宋	王怀隐，等	24.《卫生宝鉴》	明	罗天益
9.《幼幼新书》	宋	刘昉	25.《证治准绳》	明	王肯堂
10.《黄帝明堂灸经》	宋	西方子	26.《重楼玉钥》	清	郑梅涧
11.《针灸神书》	宋	琼瑶真人	27.《凌门传授铜人指穴》	清	无名氏
12.《针灸资生经》	宋	王执中	28.《针灸集成》	清	廖润鸿
13.《针经指南》	金	窦杰	29.《针灸易学》	清	李守先
14.《针经节要》	元	杜思敬	30.《针灸逢源》	清	李学川
15.《扁鹊神应针灸玉龙经》	元	王国瑞	31.《经络全书》	清	沈子禄
16.《普济方》	明	朱橚	32.《金针秘传》	民国	方慎庵

古代针灸治疗类似中风后假性球麻痹腧穴运用统计见下表。

古代针灸治疗类似中风后假性球麻痹腧穴运用统计

经脉		腧穴	频次	合计	总计
督脉	近部选穴	风府	28	86	86
		哑门	28		
		水沟	12		
		脑户	7		
		百会	6		
		前顶	3		
		囟会	2		
任脉	近部选穴	天突	28	4	54
		廉泉	19		
		承浆	7		
手阳明大肠经	近部选穴	天鼎	8	13	44
		扶突	5		
	循经取穴	合谷	29	31	
		曲池	1		
		三间	1		
手太阳小肠经	近部选穴	天窗	18	27	37
		听宫	9		
	循经取穴	后溪	9	10	
		少泽	1		
手少阴心经	循经取穴	灵道	23	34	34
		阴郄	6		
		通里	5		
手少阳三焦经	近部选穴	翳风	10	10	27
	循经取穴	支沟	10	17	
		三阳络	3		
		关冲	3		
		中渚	1		
足少阴肾经	循经取穴	涌泉	12	14	14
		然骨	1		
		太溪	1		

经脉		腧穴	频次	合计	总计
足少阳胆经	近部选穴	风池	3	8	12
		曲鬓	4		
		完骨	1		
	循经取穴	浮白	1	4	
		阳交	3		
足阳明胃经	近部选穴	大迎	1	3	11
		地仓	1		
		颊车	1		
	循经取穴	冲阳	2	8	
		内庭	2		
		足三里	2		
		丰隆	1		
		厉兑	1		
手太阴肺经	循经取穴	鱼际	5	10	10
		少商	3		
		太渊	2		
手厥阴心包经	循经取穴	间使	7	9	9
		中冲	2		
足太阳膀胱经	循经取穴	大杼	1	7	7
		通谷	3		
		昆仑	2		
		申脉	1		
足太阴脾经	循经取穴	三阴交	2	4	4
		公孙	1		
		商丘	1		
足厥阴肝经	循经取穴	期门	4	4	4
募穴		膻中	2	4	4
		鸠尾	1		
		中府	1		
背俞穴		肺俞	1	2	2
		肝俞	1		
总计		——	359	359	359

4.3.2 现代文献证据

在 CNKI（1979 ~ 2013）中以"假性球麻痹"或"延髓麻痹"为关键词进行检索，共检索到相关文献 1500 篇，剔除其中综述性和与针灸治疗无关的文献，最终命中文献 612 篇，筛除其中无法联系到原作者的文献，实际参与评价文献407篇。对命中文献进行分类并数据提取，填写数据提取表。结果如下：

现代研究文献纳入、排除情况

文献类型	中文文献			英文文献		
	检索	筛除	纳入	检索	筛除	纳入
随机对照试验	150	14	136	3	3	0
非随机同期对照试验	28	0	28	0	0	0
病例序列研究	215	12	203	9	6	0
个案报道及经验总结	14	14	0	0	0	0
总计	407	40	367	12	9	0

现代研究纳入文献

序号	作者	文献名称	出处
1	张志萍	祛风化痰针刺法治疗假性球麻痹55例临床疗效观察	湖南中医药导报，2003
2	杨国荣	头体针结合治疗假性延髓麻痹的临床观察	上海针灸杂志，2005
3	庞勇	针刺风府穴治疗假性球麻痹30例	中医杂志，2001
4	吴清明	祛风化痰针刺法治疗风痰型假性球麻痹有效性与安全性的多中心临床研究	中医药导报，2005
5	刘军	针刺治疗假性球麻痹吞咽障碍临床观察	中国针灸，1996
6	高维滨	项针治疗假性延髓麻痹的临床研究	上海针灸杂志，2000
7	刘志顺	针刺治疗中风慢性期中重度吞咽障碍临床研究	中国针灸，2002
8	刘志顺	针刺治疗假性球麻痹吞咽障碍临床研究	新中医，1998
9	吴清明	祛风化痰针刺法治疗风痰型假性球麻痹120例	中国针灸，2005
10	冯国湘	祛风化痰针法对风痰型假性球麻痹患者TCD的影响	上海针灸杂志，2005
11	刘丽莉	项针治疗假性延髓麻痹的SEP变化的动态观察	中国中医药科技，1997
12	罗平	项针配合康复训练治疗假性延髓麻痹82例	中国民间疗法，2006
13	马振河	醒脑开窍针刺法治疗假性球麻痹30例	山东中医杂志，2006
14	曾学清	针刺配合康复训练治疗脑梗塞后构音障碍30例	针灸临床杂志，2005
15	郭新民	中药配合针灸治疗中风假性球麻痹临床观察	中国医药学报，1997
16	刘书鹏	头针体针治疗脑卒中后假性球麻痹30例	中国民间疗法，2006
17	孙华	头针配合体针治疗中风假性球麻痹疗效观察	中国康复理论与实践，2006
18	靳宇	咽后壁点刺为主治疗假性延髓麻痹79例	中国针灸，1999
19	秦润笋	针刺配合康复训练治疗假性延髓性麻痹30例观察	中国实用神经疾病杂志，2006
20	沈王明	扶突穴为主治疗脑卒中假性球麻痹	针灸临床杂志，2008
21	陈晓军	靳三针治疗中风性假性球麻痹的临床研究	江苏中医药，2010
22	陈立早	舌三针联合背俞穴埋线治疗中风后假性球麻痹吞咽困难临床观察	中医药导报，2010
23	李飞	舌三针为主配合舌肌训练治疗假性球麻痹疗效观察	中医药临床杂志，2012

5 文献质量评估结论

5.1 证据概要表（evidence profile, EP）

Question: 针刺 + 基础治疗 VS 基础治疗 for 中风后假性球麻痹

Bibliography: . 针灸疗法 for 中风后假性球麻痹. Cochrane Database of Systematic Reviews [Year], Issue [Issue] .

No of studies	Quality assessment						No of patients		Effect		Quality	Importance
	Design	Risk of bias	Inconsistency	Indirectness	Imprecision	Other considerations	针刺 + 基础治疗 VS 基础治疗	Control	Relative (95% CI)	Absolute		
吞咽功能疗效评价（Follow – up 3 months）												
11	randomised trials	serious[1]	no serious inconsistency	no serious indirectness	no serious imprecision	none	504/544 (92.6%)	375/535 (70.1%)	OR 5.7 (3.9 to 8.32)	229 more per 1000 (from 200 more to 250 more)	⊕⊕⊕◯ moderate	critical
							–	74%		202 more per 1000 (from 177 more to 219 more)		
吞咽功能疗效评价 – 洼田饮水试验疗效评价（Follow – up 3 months）												
10	randomised trials	serious[1]	no serious inconsistency	no serious indirectness	no serious imprecision	none	447/482 (92.7%)	331/474 (69.8%)	OR 5.9 (3.93 to 8.86)	233 more per 1000 (from 203 more to 255 more)	⊕⊕⊕◯ moderate	critical
							–	74.2%		202 more per 1000 (from 177 more to 220 more)		
吞咽功能疗效评价 – 中风病吞咽功能疗效评定（Follow – up 3 months）												
1	randomised trials	very serious[2]	no serious inconsistency	no serious indirectness	very serious[3]	none	16/17 (94.1%)	12/16 (75%)	OR 5.33 (0.53 to 54.03)	191 more per 1000 (from 136 fewer to 244 more)	⊕◯◯◯ very low	critical
							–	75%		191 more per 1000 (from 136 fewer to 244 more)		
吞咽功能疗效评价 – 反复唾液吞咽测试疗效评价（Follow – up 3 months）												
1	randomised trials	very serious[2]	no serious inconsistency	no serious indirectness	very serious[4]	none	41/45 (91.1%)	32/45 (71.1%)	OR 4.16 (1.24 to 14)	200 more per 1000 (from 42 more to 261 more)	⊕◯◯◯ very low	critical
							–	71.1%		200 more per 1000 (from 42 more to 261 more)		

续表

No of studies	Design	Quality assessment					No of patients		Effect		Quality	Importance
		Risk of bias	Inconsistency	Indirectness	Imprecision	Other considerations	针测＋基础治疗 VS 基础治疗	Control	Relative (95% CI)	Absolute		
言语障碍疗效评价（Follow－up 1 months）												
3	randomised trials	very serious[2]	no serious inconsistency	no serious indirectness	very serious[5]	none	84/92 (91.3%)	62/91 (68.1%)	OR 5.33 (2.22 to 12.76)	238 more per 1000 (from 145 more to 283 more)	⊕○○○ very low	critical
							－	71.1%		218 more per 1000 (from 134 more to 258 more)		
言语障碍疗效评价 － 弗朗菜构音障碍评价（Follow－up 3 months）												
1	randomised trials	very serious[6]	no serious inconsistency	no serious indirectness	very serious[4]	none	28/30 (93.3%)	23/30 (76.7%)	OR 4.26 (0.81 to 22.53)	167 more per 1000 (from 40 fewer to 220 more)	⊕○○○ very low	critical
							－	76.7%		166 more per 1000 (from 40 fewer to 220 more)		
言语障碍疗效评价 － 言语功能评定（Follow－up 3 months）												
1	randomised trials	very serious[2]	no serious inconsistency	no serious indirectness	very serious[4]	none	42/45 (93.3%)	32/45 (71.1%)	OR 5.69 (1.49 to 21.66)	222 more per 1000 (from 75 more to 270 more)	⊕○○○ very low	critical
							－	71.1%		222 more per 1000 (from 75 more to 271 more)		
言语障碍疗效评价 － 中风病言语功能疗效评定（Follow－up 3 months）												
1	randomised trials	very serious[2]	no serious inconsistency	no serious indirectness	very serious[3]	none	14/17 (82.4%)	7/16 (43.8%)	OR 6 (1.22 to 29.44)	386 more per 1000 (from 49 more to 521 more)	⊕○○○ very low	critical
							－	43.8%		386 more per 1000 (from 49 more to 520 more)		
洼田氏饮水试验评分（Follow－up 3 months；Better indicated by lower values）												
3	randomised trials	serious[1]	serious[7]	no serious indirectness	no serious imprecision	none	186	186	－	SMD 1.32 higher (0.39 to 2.26 higher)	⊕⊕○○ low	critical
构音障碍积分（Follow－up 3 months；Better indicated by lower values）												
1	randomised trials	very serious[2]	no serious inconsistency	no serious indirectness	no serious imprecision	none	120	120	－	SMD 0.83 lower (1.1 to 0.57 lower)	⊕⊕○○ low	critical

1 There are unclear risk of bias.

2 There is high risk of bias.

3 Study includes relatively few patients and few events and thus has wide confidence intervals around the estimate of the effect.

4 Study has wide confidence intervals around the estimate of the effect.

5 Studies have wide confidence intervals around the estimate of the effect.

6 No explanation was provided.

7 heterogeneity exists.

Question: 祛风化痰针法 + 基础治疗 VS 假针刺 + 基础治疗 for 中风后假性球麻痹

Bibliography: : 针灸疗法 for 中风后假性球麻痹. Cochrane Database of Systematic Reviews [Year], Issue [Issue].

No of studies	Quality assessment						No of patients		Effect		Quality	Importance
	Design	Risk of bias	Inconsistency	Indirectness	Imprecision	Other considerations	祛风化痰针法 + 基础治疗 VS 假针刺 + 基础治疗	Control	Relative (95% CI)	Absolute		
中医病症疗效评价 (Follow – up 3 months)												
2	randomised trials	serious[1]	no serious in-consistency	no serious in-directness	serious[2]	none	146/160 (91.3%)	109/159 (68.6%)	OR 5.97 (2.96 to 12.04)	243 more per 1000 (from 180 more to 278 more)	⊕⊕◯◯ low	critical
							–	58.4%		309 more per 1000 (from 222 more to 360 more)		
症状体征积分 (Follow – up 3 months; Better indicated by lower values)												
1	randomised trials	serious1	no serious in-consistency	no serious in-directness	serious[3]	none	40	39	–	SMD 0.6 higher (0.15 to 1.05 higher)	⊕⊕◯◯ low	critical
洼田饮水试验评分 (Follow – up 3 months; Better indicated by lower values)												
1	randomised trials	serious1	no serious in-consistency	no serious in-directness	serious[3]	none	120	120	–	MD 0.71 higher (0.44 to 0.98 higher)	⊕⊕◯◯ low	critical

1 There is unclear risk of bias.

2 studies have wide confidence intervals around the estimate of the effect.

3 Studie has large confidence intervals around the estimate of the effect.

Question: 任督通调针刺 + 基础治疗 VS 康复治疗 + 基础治疗 for 中风后假性球麻痹

Bibliography: . 针灸疗法 for 中风后假性球麻痹. Cochrane Database of Systematic Reviews [Year], Issue [Issue].

No of studies	Quality assessment						No of patients		Effect		Quality	Importance
	Design	Risk of bias	Inconsistency	Indirectness	Imprecision	Other considerations	任督通调针刺 + 基础治疗 VS 康复治疗 + 基础治疗	Control	Relative (95% CI)	Absolute		
吞咽功能疗效评价 (Follow – up 3 months)												
2	randomised trials	very serious[1]	no serious inconsistency	no serious indirectness	very serious[2]	none	54/60 (90%) / –	38/60 (63.3%) / 63.3%	OR 5.44 (1.98 to 14.94)	270 more per 1000 (from 140 more to 329 more) / 271 more per 1000 (from 141 more to 330 more)	⊕◯◯◯ very low	critical
吞咽功能疗效评价 – 洼田饮水试验疗效评价 (Follow – up 3 months)												
1	randomised trials	very serious[1]	no serious inconsistency	no serious indirectness	very serious[3]	none	28/30 (93.3%) / –	22/30 (73.3%) / 73.3%	OR 5.09 (0.98 to 26.43)	200 more per 1000 (from 4 fewer to 253 more) / 200 more per 1000 (from 4 fewer to 253 more)	⊕◯◯◯ very low	critical
吞咽功能疗效评价 – 藤岛一郎吞咽疗效评价 (Follow – up 3 months)												
1	randomised trials	very serious[1]	no serious inconsistency	no serious indirectness	very serious[3]	none	26/30 (86.7%) / –	16/30 (53.3%) / 53.3%	OR 5.69 (1.59 to 20.33)	333 more per 1000 (from 112 more to 425 more) / 334 more per 1000 (from 112 more to 426 more)	⊕◯◯◯ very low	critical
藤岛一郎吞咽评价积分 (Follow – up 3 months; Better indicated by lower values)												
1	randomised trials	very serious[1]	no serious inconsistency	no serious indirectness	very serious[3]	none	30	30	–	SMD 1.05 lower (1.6 to 0.51 lower)	⊕◯◯◯ very low	critical

1 There are high risk of bias.

2 Studies include relatively few patients and few events and thus have wide confidence intervals around the estimate of the effect.

3 Study includes relatively few patients and few events and thus has wide confidence intervals around the estimate of the effect.

Question: 互动式针法 + 基础治疗 VS 常规针刺 + 基础治疗 for 中风后假性球麻痹

Bibliography：. 针灸疗法 for 中风后假性球麻痹. Cochrane Database of Systematic Reviews [Year], Issue [Issue].

No of studies	Quality assessment						No of patients		Effect		Quality	Importance
	Design	Risk of bias	Inconsistency	Indirectness	Imprecision	Other considerations	互动式针法+基础治疗 VS 常规针刺+基础治疗	Control	Relative (95% CI)	Absolute		
洼田饮水试验评分（Follow－up 3 months；Better indicated by lower values)												
1	randomised trials	very serious[1]	no serious inconsistency	no serious indirectness	serious[2]	none	25	25	-	SMD 0.67 higher（0.1 to 1.24 higher）	⊕○○○ very low	critical
洼田饮水试验疗效评价（Follow－up 3 months)												
2	randomised trials	very serious[1]	no serious inconsistency	no serious indirectness	very serious[3]	none	56/61（91.8%）	43/60（71.7%）	OR 4.53（1.54 to 13.31）	203 more per 1000（from 79 more to 254 more）	⊕○○○ very low	critical
							-	71.7%		203 more per 1000（from 79 more to 254 more）		

1 There are high risk of bias.

2 Study includes relatively few patients and few events.

3 studies include relatively few patients and few events and thus have wide confidence intervals around the estimate of the effect.

Question: 舌三针 + 舌肌训练 VS 假针刺 + 舌肌训练 for 中风后假性球麻痹

Bibliography：. 针灸疗法 for 中风后假性球麻痹. Cochrane Database of Systematic Reviews [Year], Issue [Issue].

No of studies	Quality assessment						No of patients		Effect		Quality	Importance
	Design	Risk of bias	Inconsistency	Indirectness	Imprecision	Other considerations	舌三针+舌肌训练 VS 假针刺+舌肌训练	Control	Relative (95% CI)	Absolute		
洼田饮水试验疗效评价（Follow－up 3 months)												
1	randomised trials	very serious[1]	no serious inconsistency	no serious indirectness	very serious[2]	none	18/20（90%）	13/20（65%）	OR 4.85（0.86 to 27.22）	250 more per 1000（from 35 fewer to 331 more）	⊕○○○ very low	critical
							-	65%		250 more per 1000（from 35 fewer to 331 more）		

1 There are high risk of bias.

2 Study includes relatively few patients and few events and thus has wide confidence intervals around the estimate of the effect.

Question：舌三针＋背俞穴埋线＋基础治疗 VS 常规针刺＋基础治疗 for 中风后假性球麻痹

Bibliography：. 针灸疗法 for 中风后假性球麻痹. Cochrane Database of Systematic Reviews [Year], Issue [Issue].

临床总疗效（Follow－up mean 3 months）

No of studies	Quality assessment						No of patients		Effect		Quality	Importance
	Design	Risk of bias	Inconsistency	Indirectness	Imprecision	Other considerations	舌三针＋背俞穴埋线＋基础治疗 VS 常规针刺＋基础治疗	Control	Relative (95% CI)	Absolute		
1	randomised trials	very serious[1]	no serious inconsistency	no serious indirectness	very serious[2]	none	26/30 (86.7%)	23/30 (76.7%)	OR 1.98 (0.51 to 7.63)	100 more per 1000 (from 140 fewer to 195 more)	⊕○○○ very low	critical
							-	76.7%		100 more per 1000 (from 140 fewer to 195 more)		

洼田饮水试验评分（Follow－up median 3 months；Better indicated by lower values）

No of studies												
1	randomised trials	very serious[1]	no serious inconsistency	no serious indirectness	serious[3]	none	30	30	-	SMD 2.35 higher (1.69 to 3.02 higher)	⊕○○○ very low	critical

1 There are high risk of bias.

2 study include relatively few patients and few events and thus has wide confidence intervals around the estimate of the effect.

3 Study includes relatively few patients and few events.

Question: 电针 + 基础治疗 VS 针刺 + 基础治疗 for 中风后假性球麻痹

Bibliography: . 针灸疗法 for 中风后假性球麻痹. Cochrane Database of Systematic Reviews [Year], Issue [Issue].

No of studies	Quality assessment						No of patients		Effect		Quality	Importance
	Design	Risk of bias	Inconsistency	Indirectness	Imprecision	Other considerations	电针 + 基础治疗 VS 针刺 + 基础治疗	Control	Relative (95% CI)	Absolute		

各项指标疗效评价 (Follow – up 3 months)

No of studies	Design	Risk of bias	Inconsistency	Indirectness	Imprecision	Other considerations	电针 + 基础治疗 VS 针刺 + 基础治疗	Control	Relative (95% CI)	Absolute	Quality	Importance
1	randomised trials	serious[1]	no serious inconsistency	no serious indirectness	very serious[2]	none	26/30 (86.7%)	18/30 (60%)	OR 4.33 (1.2 to 15.61)	267 more per 1000 (from 43 more to 359 more)	⊕○○○ very low	critical
							–	60%		267 more per 1000 (from 43 more to 359 more)		

各项指标评价积分 (Better indicated by lower values)

No of studies	Design	Risk of bias	Inconsistency	Indirectness	Imprecision	Other considerations	电针 + 基础治疗 VS 针刺 + 基础治疗	Control	Relative (95% CI)	Absolute	Quality	Importance
1	randomised trials	serious[1]	no serious inconsistency	no serious indirectness	serious[3]	none	30	30	–	SMD 0.9 lower (1.43 to 0.37 lower)	⊕⊕○○ low	critical

1 There are unclear risk of bias.

2 Study includes relatively few patients and few events and thus has wide confidence intervals around the estimate of the effect.

3 Study includes relatively few patients and few events.

Question: 舌下针 + 基础治疗 VS 基础治疗 for 中风后假性球麻痹

Bibliography: . 针灸疗法 for 中风后假性球麻痹. Cochrane Database of Systematic Reviews [Year], Issue [Issue] .

No of studies	Quality assessment						No of patients		Effect		Quality	Importance
	Design	Risk of bias	Inconsistency	Indirectness	Imprecision	Other considerations	舌下针 + 基础治疗 VS 基础治疗	Control	Relative (95% CI)	Absolute		
各项指标评价积分 (Follow – up 3 months; Better indicated by lower values)												
1	randomised trials	serious[1]	serious[2]	no serious in-directness	serious[3]	none	150	150	–	SMD 0.32 lower (0.76 lower to 0.12 higher)	⊕○○○ very low	critical
各项指标评价积分 – 总症状积分 (Follow – up 3 months; Better indicated by lower values)												
1	randomised trials	serious[1]	no serious in-consistency	no serious in-directness	serious[3]	none	30	30	–	SMD 0.42 higher (0.09 lower to 0.93 higher)	⊕⊕○○ low	critical
各项指标评价积分 – 构音障碍 (Follow – up 3 months; Better indicated by lower values)												
1	randomised trials	serious[1]	no serious in-consistency	no serious in-directness	serious[3]	none	30	30	–	SMD 0.84 lower (1.37 to 0.31 lower)	⊕⊕○○ low	critical
各项指标评价积分 – 吞咽障碍 (Follow – up 3 months; Better indicated by lower values)												
1	randomised trials	serious[1]	no serious in-consistency	no serious in-directness	serious[3]	none	30	30	–	SMD 0.5 lower (1.02 lower to 0.01 higher)	⊕⊕○○ low	critical
各项指标评价积分 – 舌体运动 (Follow – up 3 months; Better indicated by lower values)												
1	randomised trials	serious[1]	no serious in-consistency	no serious in-directness	serious[3]	none	30	30	–	SMD 0.63 lower (1.15 to 0.11 lower)	⊕⊕○○ low	critical
各项指标评价积分 – 情感状态 (Follow – up 3 months; Better indicated by lower values)												
1	randomised trials	serious[1]	no serious in-consistency	no serious in-directness	serious[3]	none	30	30	–	SMD 0.07 lower (0.58 lower to 0.43 higher)	⊕⊕○○ low	critical

1 There are unclear risk of bias.

2 heterogeneity exists

3 Study includes relatively few patients and few events.

Question: 项针 + 基础治疗 VS 基础治疗 for 中风后假性球麻痹

Bibliography: . 针灸疗法 for 中风后假性球麻痹. Cochrane Database of Systematic Reviews [Year], Issue [Issue] .

No of studies	Quality assessment						No of patients		Effect		Quality	Importance
	Design	Risk of bias	Inconsistency	Indirectness	Imprecision	Other considerations	项针 + 基础治疗 VS 基础治疗	Control	Relative (95% CI)	Absolute		
洼田饮水试验疗效评价 (Follow – up 3 months)												
1	randomised trials	serious[1]	no serious inconsistency	no serious indirectness	serious[2]	none	38/46 (82.6%) / -	29/46 (63%) / 63%	OR 2.78 (1.06 to 7.34)	195 more per 1000 (from 13 more to 296 more) / 196 more per 1000 (from 13 more to 296 more)	⊕⊕◯◯ low	critical
大西幸子吞咽功能疗效评价 (Follow – up 3 months)												
2	randomised trials	very serious[3]	no serious inconsistency	no serious indirectness	serious[4]	none	121/128 (94.5%) / -	93/128 (72.7%) / 71.3%	OR 6.66 (2.8 to 15.8)	220 more per 1000 (from 155 more to 250 more) / 230 more per 1000 (from 161 more to 262 more)	⊕◯◯◯ very low	critical
大西幸子言语功能疗效评价 (Follow – up 3 months)												
2	randomised trials	very serious[3]	no serious inconsistency	no serious indirectness	serious[4]	none	109/128 (85.2%) / -	68/128 (53.1%) / 55%	OR 4.58 (1.79 to 11.71)	307 more per 1000 (from 139 more to 399 more) / 298 more per 1000 (from 136 more to 385 more)	⊕◯◯◯ very low	critical

1 There are unclear risk of bias.
2 Study has wide confidence intervals around the estimate of the effect.
3 There are high risk of bias.
4 Studies have wide confidence intervals around the estimate of the effect.

Question：颈项针 + 基础治疗 VS 舌三针 + 基础治疗 for 中风后假性球麻痹

Bibliography：．针灸疗法 for 中风后假性球麻痹．Cochrane Database of Systematic Reviews [Year], Issue [Issue].

中医病症疗效评价（Follow－up 3 months）

No of studies	Quality assessment						No of patients		Effect		Quality	Importance
	Design	Risk of bias	Inconsistency	Indirectness	Imprecision	Other considerations	颈项针 + 基础治疗 VS 舌三针 + 基础治疗	Control	Relative (95% CI)	Absolute		
1	randomised trials	very serious[1]	no serious inconsistency	no serious indirectness	serious[2]	none	54/60 (90%)	49/60 (81.7%)	OR 2.02 (0.69 to 5.87)	83 more per 1000 (from 62 fewer to 146 more)	⊕○○○ very low	critical
							-	81.7%		83 more per 1000 (from 62 fewer to 146 more)		

中医病症状体征积分（Follow－up 3 months; Better indicated by lower values）

No of studies	Quality assessment						No of patients		Effect		Quality	Importance
1	randomised trials	very serious[1]	no serious inconsistency	no serious indirectness	no serious imprecision[2]	none	60	60	-	SMD 0.36 higher (0 to 0.72 higher)	⊕⊕○○ low	critical

1 There are high risk of bias.

2 Study has wide confidence intervals around the estimate of the effect

Question：醒脑开窍针刺法 + 基础治疗 VS 常规针刺法 + 基础治疗 for 中风后假性球麻痹

Bibliography：．针灸疗法 for 中风后假性球麻痹．Cochrane Database of Systematic Reviews [Year], Issue [Issue].

中医病症疗效评价（Follow－up 3 months）

No of studies	Quality assessment						No of patients		Effect		Quality	Importance
	Design	Risk of bias	Inconsistency	Indirectness	Imprecision	Other considerations	醒脑开窍针刺法 + 基础治疗 VS 常规针刺法 + 基础治疗	Control	Relative (95% CI)	Absolute		
2	randomised trials	serious[1]	no serious inconsistency	no serious indirectness	serious[2]	none	83/87 (95.4%)	68/83 (81.9%)	OR 4.56 (1.45 to 14.4)	135 more per 1000 (from 49 more to 166 more)	⊕⊕⊕○ low	important
							-	81.9%		135 more per 1000 (from 49 more to 166 more)		

1 There are unclear risk of bias.

2 2 studies has wide confidence intervals around the estimate of the effect

Question: 醒脑开窍针法 + 基础治疗 VS 基础治疗 for 中风后假性球麻痹

Bibliography:. 针灸疗法 for 中风后假性球麻痹. Cochrane Database of Systematic Reviews [Year], Issue [Issue].

No of studies	Quality assessment						No of patients		Effect		Quality	Importance
	Design	Risk of bias	Inconsistency	Indirectness	Imprecision	Other considerations	醒脑开窍针法 + 基础治疗 VS 基础治疗	Control	Relative (95% CI)	Absolute		

吞咽功能疗效评价 (Follow – up 3 months)

| 1 | randomised trials | very serious[1] | no serious inconsistency | no serious indirectness | serious[2] | none | 64/68 (94.1%) | 31/52 (59.6%) | OR 10.84 (3.42 to 34.3) | 345 more per 1000 (from 239 more to 384 more) | ⊕○○○ very low | critical |
| | | | | | | | – | 59.6% | | 345 more per 1000 (from 239 more to 385 more) | | |

洼田氏饮水试验评分 (Follow – up 3 months; Better indicated by lower values)

| 1 | randomised trials | very serious[1] | no serious inconsistency | no serious indirectness | no serious imprecision[2] | none | 68 | 52 | – | SMD 0.87 higher (0.49 to 1.25 higher) | ⊕⊕○○ low | critical |

1 There are high risk of bias.
2 Study has wide confidence intervals around the estimate of the effect

Question: 舌咽针 + 基础疗法 VS 基础疗法 for 中风后假性球麻痹

Bibliography: . 针灸疗法 for 中风后假性球麻痹. Cochrane Database of Systematic Reviews [Year], Issue [Issue].

临床症状疗效评价 (Follow – up 3 months)

No of studies	Quality assessment						No of patients		Effect		Quality	Importance
	Design	Risk of bias	Inconsistency	Indirectness	Imprecision	Other considerations	舌咽针 + 基础疗法 VS 基础疗法	Control	Relative (95% CI)	Absolute		
1	randomised trials	serious[1]	no serious inconsistency	no serious indirectness	very serious[2]	none	29/30 (96.7%)	26/30 (86.7%)	OR 4.46 (0.47 to 42.51)	100 more per 1000 (from 113 fewer to 130 more)	⊕○○○ very low	critical
							–	86.7%		100 more per 1000 (from 113 fewer to 129 more)		

洼田饮水试验疗效评价 (Follow – up 3 months)

No of studies	Quality assessment						No of patients		Effect		Quality	Importance
	Design	Risk of bias	Inconsistency	Indirectness	Imprecision	Other considerations	舌咽针 + 基础疗法 VS 基础疗法	Control	Relative (95% CI)	Absolute		
1	randomised trials	serious[1]	no serious inconsistency	no serious indirectness	very serious[2]	none	27/30 (90%)	22/30 (73.3%)	OR 3.27 (0.77 to 13.83)	167 more per 1000 (from 54 fewer to 241 more)	⊕○○○ very low	critical
							–	73.3%		167 more per 1000 (from 54 fewer to 241 more)		

1 There are unclear risk of bias.

2 Study includes relatively few patients and few events and thus has wide confidence intervals around the estimate of the effect

Question: 舌咽针 + 基础治疗 VS 常规针刺 + 基础治疗 for 中风后假性球麻痹

Bibliography: . 针灸疗法 for 中风后假性球麻痹. Cochrane Database of Systematic Reviews [Year], Issue [Issue].

洼田饮水试验疗效评价 (Follow – up 3 months)

No of studies	Quality assessment						No of patients		Effect		Quality	Importance
	Design	Risk of bias	Inconsistency	Indirectness	Imprecision	Other considerations	舌咽针 + 基础治疗 VS 常规针刺 + 基础治疗	Control	Relative (95% CI)	Absolute		
2	randomised trials	serious[1]	no serious inconsistency	no serious indirectness	very serious[2]	none	56/61 (91.8%)	43/60 (71.7%)	OR 4.53 (1.54 to 13.31)	203 more per 1000 (from 79 more to 254 more)	⊕○○○ very low	critical
							–	71.7%		203 more per 1000 (from 79 more to 254 more)		

1 There are unclear risk of bias.

2 Studies include relatively few patients and few events and thus have wide confidence intervals around the estimate of the effect.

Question：穴位注射 + 基础治疗 VS 基础治疗 for 中风后假性球麻痹

Bibliography：. 针灸疗法 for 中风后假性球麻痹 . Cochrane Database of Systematic Reviews [Year], Issue [Issue] .

临床症状疗效评价 (Follow – up 3 months)

No of studies	Design	Risk of bias	Inconsistency	Indirectness	Imprecision	Other considerations	穴位注射 + 基础治疗 VS 基础治疗	Control	Relative (95% CI)	Absolute	Quality	Importance
				Quality assessment			No of patients		Effect			
2	randomised trials	very serious[1]	no serious inconsistency	no serious indirectness	serious[2]	none	175/182 (96.2%)	136/185 (73.5%)	OR 9.7 (4.22 to 22.27)	229 more per 1000 (from 186 more to 249 more)	⊕○○○ very low	critical
							–	74%		225 more per 1000 (from 183 more to 244 more)		

1 There are high risk of bias.
2 studies have wide confidence intervals around the estimate of the effect

Question：穴位注射 + 基础治疗 VS 常规针刺 + 基础治疗 for 中风后假性球麻痹

Bibliography：. 针灸疗法 for 中风后假性球麻痹 . Cochrane Database of Systematic Reviews [Year], Issue [Issue] .

洼田饮水试验疗效评价 (Follow – up 3 months)

No of studies	Design	Risk of bias	Inconsistency	Indirectness	Imprecision	Other considerations	穴位注射 + 基础治疗 VS 常规针刺 + 基础治疗	Control	Relative (95% CI)	Absolute	Quality	Importance
				Quality assessment			No of patients		Effect			
1	randomised trials	very serious1	no serious inconsistency	no serious indirectness	very serious[2,3]	none	28/30 (93.3%)	21/30 (70%)	OR 6 (1.17 to 30.72)	233 more per 1000 (from 32 more to 286 more)	⊕○○○ very low	critical
							–	70%		233 more per 1000 (from 32 more to 286 more)		

1 There are high risk of bias.
2 No explanation was provided.
3 Study includes relatively few patients and few events and thus has wide confidence intervals around the estimate of the effect.

Question: 耳针 + 常规针刺 + 基础疗法 VS 常规针刺 + 基础疗法 for 中风后假性球麻痹

Bibliography:. 针灸疗法 for 中风后假性球麻痹. Cochrane Database of Systematic Reviews [Year], Issue [Issue].

洼田饮水试验疗效评价 (Follow – up 3 months)

No of studies	Quality assessment						No of patients		Effect		Quality	Importance
	Design	Risk of bias	Inconsistency	Indirectness	Imprecision	Other considerations	耳针 + 常规针刺 + 基础疗法 VS 常规针刺 + 基础疗法	Control	Relative (95% CI)	Absolute		
1	randomised trials	very serious[1]	no serious inconsistency	no serious indirectness	very serious[2]	none	11/14 (78.6%)	9/14 (64.3%)	OR 2.04 (0.38 to 10.94)	143 more per 1000 (from 237 fewer to 309 more)	⊕○○○ very low	critical
							-	64.3%		143 more per 1000 (from 237 fewer to 309 more)		

洼田饮水试验评分 (Follow – up 3 months; Better indicated by lower values)

No of studies							No of patients		Effect		Quality	Importance
1	randomised trials	very serious[1]	no serious inconsistency	no serious indirectness	very serious[2]	none	14	14	-	SMD 2.85 higher (1.75 to 3.94 higher)	⊕○○○ very low	critical

1 There are high risk of bias.　　2 Study includes relatively few patients and few events and thus has wide confidence intervals around the estimate of the effect.

Question: 康复训练 + 针刺 + 基础治疗 VS 针刺 + 基础治疗 for 中风后假性球麻痹

Bibliography:. 针灸疗法 for 中风后假性球麻痹. Cochrane Database of Systematic Reviews [Year], Issue [Issue].

构音障碍疗效评价 (Follow – up 3 months)

No of studies	Quality assessment						No of patients		Effect		Quality	Importance
	Design	Risk of bias	Inconsistency	Indirectness	Imprecision	Other considerations	康复训练 + 针刺 + 基础治疗 VS 针刺 + 基础治疗	Control	Relative (95% CI)	Absolute		
1	randomised trials	very serious[1]	no serious inconsistency	no serious indirectness	serious[2]	none	33/42 (78.6%)	21/42 (50%)	OR 3.67 (1.41 to 9.51)	286 more per 1000 (from 85 more to 405 more)	⊕○○○ very low	critical
							-	50%		286 more per 1000 (from 85 more to 405 more)		

洼田饮水试验评分 (Follow – up 3 months; Better indicated by lower values)

No of studies							No of patients		Effect		Quality	Importance
1	randomised trials	very serious[1]	no serious inconsistency	no serious indirectness	no serious imprecision[2]	none	48	48	-	SMD 0.19 higher (0.21 lower to 0.59 higher)	⊕⊕○○ low	critical

1 There are high risk of bias.　　2 Study has wide confidence intervals around the estimate of the effect.

Question：靳三针＋基础治疗 VS 常规针刺＋基础治疗 for 中风后假性球麻痹

Bibliography：. 针灸疗法 for 中风后假性球麻痹. Cochrane Database of Systematic Reviews [Year], Issue [Issue].

症状体征疗效评价（Follow－up 3 months)

No of studies	Quality assessment						No of patients		Effect		Quality	Importance
	Design	Risk of bias	Inconsistency	Indirectness	Imprecision	Other considerations	靳三针＋基础治疗 VS 常规针刺＋基础治疗	Control	Relative (95% CI)	Absolute		
1	randomised trials	very serious[1]	no serious inconsistency	no serious indirectness	very serious[2]	none	35/40 (87.5%)	35/40 (87.5%)	OR 1 (0.27 to 3.76)	0 fewer per 1000（from 221 fewer to 88 more)	⊕◯◯◯ very low	critical
							-	87.5%		0 fewer per 1000（from 221 fewer to 88 more)		

症状体征积分评价（Follow－up 3 months; Better indicated by lower values)

No of studies	Design	Risk of bias	Inconsistency	Indirectness	Imprecision	Other considerations	Treatment	Control	Relative (95% CI)	Absolute	Quality	Importance
1	randomised trials	very serious[1]	no serious inconsistency	no serious indirectness	serious[3]	none	40	40	–	SMD 0.76 higher (0.31 to 1.22 higher)	⊕◯◯◯ very low	critical

1 There are high risk of bias.
2 Study includes relatively few patients and few events and thus has wide confidence intervals around the estimate of the effect
3 Study includes relatively few patients and few events.

Question：耳三针＋基础治疗 VS 基础治疗 for 中风后假性球麻痹

Bibliography：. 针灸疗法 for 中风后假性球麻痹. Cochrane Database of Systematic Reviews [Year], Issue [Issue].

洼田饮水试验评分（Follow－up 3 months; Better indicated by lower values)

No of studies	Quality assessment						No of patients		Effect		Quality	Importance
	Design	Risk of bias	Inconsistency	Indirectness	Imprecision	Other considerations	耳三针＋基础治疗 VS 基础治疗	Control	Relative (95% CI)	Absolute		
1	randomised trials	very serious[1]	no serious inconsistency	no serious indirectness	serious[2]	none	40	40	–	SMD 0.63 higher (0.18 to 1.08 higher)	⊕◯◯◯ very low	critical

藤岛一郎吞咽障碍评分（Follow－up 3 months; Better indicated by lower values)

No of studies	Design	Risk of bias	Inconsistency	Indirectness	Imprecision	Other considerations	Treatment	Control	Relative (95% CI)	Absolute	Quality	Importance
1	randomised trials	very serious[1]	no serious inconsistency	no serious indirectness	serious[2]	none	40	40	–	SMD 0.43 lower (0.88 lower to 0.01 higher)	⊕◯◯◯ very low	critical

1 There are high risk of bias.
2 Study includes relatively few patients and few events.

Question: 深刺人迎穴＋常规针刺＋基础治疗 VS 常规针刺＋基础治疗 for 中风后假性球麻痹

Bibliography：. 针灸疗法 for 中风后假性球麻痹. Cochrane Database of Systematic Reviews [Year], Issue [Issue].

No of studies	Quality assessment						No of patients		Effect		Quality	Importance
	Design	Risk of bias	Inconsistency	Indirectness	Imprecision	Other considerations	深刺人迎穴 ＋常规针刺 ＋基础治疗 VS 常规针刺 ＋基础治疗	Control	Relative (95% CI)	Absolute		

洼田氏饮水试验疗效评价（Follow – up 3 months）

No of studies	Design	Risk of bias	Inconsistency	Indirectness	Imprecision	Other considerations	深刺人迎穴 ＋常规针刺 ＋基础治疗 VS 常规针刺 ＋基础治疗	Control	Relative (95% CI)	Absolute	Quality	Importance
1	randomised trials	serious[1]	no serious inconsistency	no serious indirectness	serious[2]	none	56/60 (93.3%)	45/60 (75%)	OR 4.67 (1.45 to 15.05)	183 more per 1000 (from 63 more to 228 more)	⊕⊕⊕○○ low	critical
							–	75%		183 more per 1000 (from 63 more to 228 more)		

洼田氏饮水试验评分（Follow – up 3 months; Better indicated by lower values）

No of studies	Design	Risk of bias	Inconsistency	Indirectness	Imprecision	Other considerations	深刺人迎穴 ＋常规针刺 ＋基础治疗 VS 常规针刺 ＋基础治疗	Control	Relative (95% CI)	Absolute	Quality	Importance
1	randomised trials	serious[1]	no serious inconsistency	no serious indirectness	serious[2]	none	60	60	–	SMD 2.41 higher (1.93 to 2.88 higher)	⊕⊕⊕○○ low	critical

1 There are unclear risk of bias.

2 Study has wide confidence intervals around the estimate of the effect.

Question：针刺扶突穴＋头针＋基础治疗 VS 头针＋基础治疗 for 中风后假性球麻痹

Bibliography：．针灸疗法 for 中风后假性球麻痹．Cochrane Database of Systematic Reviews［Year］，Issue［Issue］．

临床症状疗效评价（Follow－up 3 months）

No of studies	Quality assessment						No of patients		Effect		Quality	Importance
	Design	Risk of bias	Inconsistency	Indirectness	Imprecision	Other considerations	针刺扶突穴＋头针＋基础治疗 VS 头针＋基础治疗	Control	Relative (95% CI)	Absolute		
1	randomised trials	serious[1]	no serious inconsistency	no serious indirectness	serious[2]	none	70/75 (93.3%)	65/75 (86.7%)	OR 2.15 (0.7 to 6.64)	67 more per 1000 (from 47 fewer to 111 more)	⊕⊕◯◯ low	critical
							-	86.7%		66 more per 1000 (from 47 fewer to 110 more)		

洼田饮水试验疗效评价（Follow－up 3 months）

No of studies	Quality assessment						No of patients		Effect		Quality	Importance
	Design	Risk of bias	Inconsistency	Indirectness	Imprecision	Other considerations	针刺扶突穴＋头针＋基础治疗 VS 头针＋基础治疗	Control	Relative (95% CI)	Absolute		
1	randomised trials	serious[1]	no serious inconsistency	no serious indirectness	serious[2]	none	69/75 (92%)	58/75 (77.3%)	OR 3.37 (1.25 to 9.11)	147 more per 1000 (from 37 more to 195 more)	⊕⊕◯◯ low	critical
							-	77.3%		147 more per 1000 (from 37 more to 196 more)		

1 There are unclear risk of bias.

2 Study has wide confidence intervals around the estimate of the effect.

5.2 结果汇总表 (the summary of findings table, SoFs table)

针刺 + 基础治疗 VS 基础治疗 for 中风后假性球麻痹

Patient or population: patients with 中风后假性球麻痹

Intervention: 针刺 + 基础治疗 VS 基础治疗

Outcomes	Illustrative comparative risks* (95% CI)		Relative effect (95% CI)	No of Participants (studies)	Quality of the evidence (GRADE)	Comments
	Assumed risk	Corresponding risk				
	Control	针刺 + 基础治疗 VS 基础治疗				
吞咽功能疗效评价 Follow – up: 3 months	Study population		OR 5.7 (3.9 to 8.32)	1079 (11 studies)	⊕⊕⊕⊝ moderate[1]	.
	701 per 1000	930 per 1000 (901 to 951)				
	Moderate					
	740 per 1000	942 per 1000 (917 to 959)				
吞咽功能疗效评价 – 洼田饮水试验疗效评价 Follow – up: 3 months	Study population		OR 5.9 (3.93 to 8.86)	956 (10 studies)	⊕⊕⊕⊝ moderate[1]	
	698 per 1000	932 per 1000 (901 to 954)				
	Moderate					
	742 per 1000	944 per 1000 (919 to 962)				
吞咽功能疗效评价 – 中风病吞咽功能疗效评定 Follow – up: 3 months	Study population		OR 5.33 (0.53 to 54.03)	33 (1 study)	⊕⊝⊝⊝ very low[2,3]	
	750 per 1000	941 per 1000 (614 to 994)				
	Moderate					
	750 per 1000	941 per 1000 (614 to 994)				

续表

Outcomes	Assumed risk	Corresponding risk	Relative effect (95% CI)	No of Participants (studies)	Quality of the evidence (GRADE)
吞咽功能疗效评价 – 反复唾液吞咽测试疗效评价 Follow-up: 3 months	Study population 711 per 1000	911 per 1000 (753 to 972)	OR 4.16 (1.24 to 14)	90 (1 study)	⊕⊕⊕⊖ very low[2,4]
	Moderate 711 per 1000	911 per 1000 (753 to 972)			
言语障碍疗效评价 Follow-up: 1 months	Study population 681 per 1000	919 per 1000 (826 to 965)	OR 5.33 (2.22 to 12.76)	183 (3 studies)	⊕⊕⊕⊖ very low[2,5]
	Moderate 711 per 1000	929 per 1000 (845 to 969)			
言语障碍疗效评价 – 弗朗菜构音障碍评价 Follow-up: 3 months	Study population 767 per 1000	933 per 1000 (727 to 987)	OR 4.26 (0.81 to 22.53)	60 (1 study)	⊕⊕⊕⊖ very low[4,6]
	Moderate 767 per 1000	933 per 1000 (727 to 987)			
言语障碍疗效评价 – 言语功能评定 Follow-up: 3 months	Study population 711 per 1000	933 per 1000 (786 to 982)	OR 5.69 (1.49 to 21.66)	90 (1 study)	⊕⊕⊕⊖ very low[2,4]
	Moderate 711 per 1000	933 per 1000 (786 to 982)			

续表

Outcomes	Illustrative comparative risks* (95% CI)		Relative effect (95% CI)	No of Participants (studies)	Quality of the evidence (GRADE)
	Assumed risk	Corresponding risk			
言语障碍疗效评价 - 中风病言语功能疗效评定 Follow - up: 3 months	Study population 438 per 1000	824 per 1000 (487 to 958)	OR 6 (1.22 to 29.44)	33 (1 study)	⊕◯◯◯ very low[2,3]
	Moderate 438 per 1000	824 per 1000 (487 to 958)			
洼田饮水试验评分 Follow - up: 3 months		The mean 洼田饮水试验评分 in the intervention groups was 1.32 standard deviations higher (0.39 to 2.26 higher)	SMD 1.32 (0.39 to 2.26)	372 (3 studies)	⊕⊕◯◯ low[1,7]
构音障碍积分 Follow - up: 3 months		The mean 构音障碍积分 in the intervention groups was 0.83 standard deviations lower (1.1 to 0.57 lower)	SMD -0.83 (-1.1 to -0.57)	240 (1 study)	⊕⊕◯◯ low[2]

* The basis for the assumed risk (e. g. the median control group risk across studies) is provided in footnotes. The corresponding risk (and its 95% confidence interval) is based on the assumed risk in the comparison group and the relative effect of the intervention (and its 95% CI).

CI: Confidence interval; OR: Odds ratio.

GRADE Working Group grades of evidence

High quality: Further research is very unlikely to change our confidence in the estimate of effect.

Moderate quality: Further research is likely to have an important impact on our confidence in the estimate of effect and may change the estimate.

Low quality: Further research is very likely to have an important impact on our confidence in the estimate of effect and is likely to change the estimate.

Very low quality: We are very uncertain about the estimate.

1 There are unclear risk of bias.

2 There is high risk of bias.

3 Study includes relatively few patients and few events and thus has wide confidence intervals around the estimate of the effect.

4 Study has wide confidence intervals around the estimate of the effect.

5 Studies have wide confidence intervals around the estimate of the effect.

6 No explanation was provided.

7 heterogeneity exists.

祛风化痰针法 + 基础治疗 VS 假针刺 + 基础治疗 for 中风后假性球麻痹

Patient or population: patients with 中风后假性球麻痹 Intervention: 祛风化痰针法 + 基础治疗 VS 假针刺 + 基础治疗

Outcomes	Illustrative comparative risks* (95% CI)		Relative effect (95% CI)	No of Participants (studies)	Quality of the evidence (GRADE)	Comments
	Assumed risk Control	Corresponding risk 祛风化痰针法 + 基础治疗 VS 假针刺 + 基础治疗				
	Study population					
中医病症疗效评价 Follow－up: 3 months	686 per 1000	929 per 1000 (866 to 963)	OR 5.97 (2.96 to 12.04)	319 (2 studies)	⊕⊕⊝⊝ low[1,2]	
	Moderate					
	584 per 1000	893 per 1000 (806 to 944)				
症状体征积分 Follow－up: 3 months		The mean 症状体征积分 in the intervention groups was 0.6 standard deviations higher (0.15 to 1.05 higher)		79 (1 study)	⊕⊕⊝⊝ low[1,3]	SMD 0.6 (0.15 to 1.05)
洼田饮水试验评分 Follow－up: 3 months		The mean 洼田饮水试验评分 in the intervention groups was 0.71 higher (0.44 to 0.98 higher)		240 (1 study)	⊕⊕⊝⊝ low[1,3]	

* The basis for the assumed risk（e. g. the median control group risk across studies）is provided in footnotes. The corresponding risk（and its 95% confidence interval）is based on the assumed risk in the comparison group and the relative effect of the intervention（and its 95% CI）.

CI: Confidence interval; OR: Odds ratio.

GRADE Working Group grades of evidence

High quality: Further research is very unlikely to change our confidence in the estimate of effect.

Moderate quality: Further research is likely to have an important impact on our confidence in the estimate of effect and may change the estimate.

Low quality: Further research is very likely to have an important impact on our confidence in the estimate of effect and is likely to change the estimate.

Very low quality: We are very uncertain about the estimate.

1 There is unclear risk of bias.

2 studies have wide confidence intervals around the estimate of the effect.

3 Studie has large confidence intervals around the estimate of the effect.

任督通调针刺 + 基础治疗 VS 康复治疗 + 基础治疗 for 中风后假性球麻痹

Patient or population: patients with 中风后假性球麻痹
Intervention: 任督通调针刺 + 基础治疗 + 基础治疗 VS 康复治疗 + 基础治疗

Outcomes	Illustrative comparative risks* (95% CI) Assumed risk — Control	Corresponding risk — 任督通调针刺 + 基础治疗 VS 康复治疗 + 基础治疗	Relative effect (95% CI)	No of Participants (studies)	Quality of the evidence (GRADE)	Comments
吞咽功能疗效评价 Follow-up: 3 months	Study population 633 per 1000	904 per 1000 (774 to 963)	OR 5.44 (1.98 to 14.94)	120 (2 studies)	⊕⊝⊝⊝ very low[1,2]	
	Moderate 633 per 1000	904 per 1000 (774 to 963)				
吞咽功能疗效评价 - 洼田饮水试验疗效评价 Follow-up: 3 months	Study population 733 per 1000	933 per 1000 (729 to 986)	OR 5.09 (0.98 to 26.43)	60 (1 study)	⊕⊝⊝⊝ very low[1,3]	
	Moderate 733 per 1000	933 per 1000 (729 to 986)				
吞咽功能疗效评价 - 藤岛一郎吞咽疗效评价 Follow-up: 3 months	Study population 867 per 1000	533 per 1000 (645 to 959)	OR 5.69 (1.59 to 20.33)	60 (1 study)	⊕⊝⊝⊝ very low[1,3]	
	Moderate 867 per 1000	533 per 1000 (645 to 959)				
藤岛一郎吞咽评价积分 Follow-up: 3 months		The mean 藤岛一郎吞咽评价积分 in the intervention groups was 1.05 standard deviations lower (1.6 to 0.51 lower)		60 (1 study)	⊕⊝⊝⊝ very low[1,3]	SMD － 1.05 (－1.6 to －0.51)

续表

* The basis for the assumed risk (e. g. the median control group risk across studies) is provided in footnotes. The corresponding risk (and its 95% confidence interval) is based on the assumed risk in the comparison group and the relative effect of the intervention (and its 95% CI).

CI: Confidence interval; OR: Odds ratio.

GRADE Working Group grades of evidence

High quality: Further research is very unlikely to change our confidence in the estimate of effect.

Moderate quality: Further research is likely to have an important impact on our confidence in the estimate of effect and may change the estimate.

Low quality: Further research is very likely to have an important impact on our confidence in the estimate of effect and is likely to change the estimate.

Very low quality: We are very uncertain about the estimate.

1 There are high risk of bias.

2 Studies include relatively few patients and few events and thus have wide confidence intervals around the estimate of the effect.

3 Study includes relatively few patients and few events and thus has wide confidence intervals around the estimate of the effect.

互动式针法 + 基础治疗 VS 常规针刺 + 基础治疗 for 中风后假性球麻痹

Patient or population: patients with 中风后假性球麻痹
Intervention: 互动式针法 + 基础治疗 VS 常规针刺 + 基础治疗

Outcomes	Illustrative comparative risks* (95% CI)		Relative effect (95% CI)	No of Participants (studies)	Quality of the evidence (GRADE)	Comments
	Assumed risk Control	Corresponding risk 互动式针法 + 基础治疗 VS 常规针刺 + 基础治疗				
洼田饮水试验评分 Follow – up: 3 months		The mean 洼田氏饮水试验评分 in the intervention groups was 0.67 standard deviations higher (0.1 to 1.24 higher)		50 (1 study)	⊕⊖⊖⊖ very low[1,2]	SMD 0.67 (0.1 to 1.24)
洼田饮水试验疗效评价 Follow – up: 3 months	Study population					
	717 per 1000	920 per 1000 (796 to 971)	OR 4.53 (1.54 to 13.31)	121 (2 studies)	⊕⊖⊖⊖ very low[1,3]	
	Moderate					
	717 per 1000	920 per 1000 (796 to 971)				

* The basis for the assumed risk (e. g. the median control group risk across studies) is provided in footnotes. The corresponding risk (and its 95% confidence interval) is based on the assumed risk in the comparison group and the relative effect of the intervention (and its 95% CI).
CI: Confidence interval; OR: Odds ratio.

GRADE Working Group grades of evidence
High quality: Further research is very unlikely to change our confidence in the estimate of effect.
Moderate quality: Further research is likely to have an important impact on our confidence in the estimate of effect and may change the estimate.
Low quality: Further research is very likely to have an important impact on our confidence in the estimate of effect and is likely to change the estimate.
Very low quality: We are very uncertain about the estimate.

1 There are high risk of bias.
2 Study includes relatively few patients and few events.
3 studies include relatively few patients and few events and thus have wide confidence intervals around the estimate of the effect.

舌三针+舌肌训练 VS 假针刺+舌肌训练 for 中风后假性球麻痹

Patient or population: patients with 中风后假性球麻痹
Intervention: 舌三针+舌肌训练 VS 假针刺+舌肌训练

Outcomes	Illustrative comparative risks* (95% CI)		Relative effect (95% CI)	No of Participants (studies)	Quality of the evidence (GRADE)	Comments
	Assumed risk	Corresponding risk				
	Control	舌三针+舌肌训练 VS 假针刺+舌肌训练				
	Study population					
洼田饮水试验疗效评价 Follow-up: 3 months	650 per 1000	900 per 1000 (615 to 981)	OR 4.85 (0.86 to 27.22)	40 (1 study)	⊕⊝⊝⊝ very low[1,2]	
	Moderate					
	650 per 1000	900 per 1000 (615 to 981)				

* The basis for the assumed risk (e.g. the median control group risk across studies) is provided in footnotes. The corresponding risk (and its 95% confidence interval) is based on the assumed risk in the comparison group and the relative effect of the intervention (and its 95% CI).
CI: Confidence interval; OR: Odds ratio.

GRADE Working Group grades of evidence
High quality: Further research is very unlikely to change our confidence in the estimate of effect.
Moderate quality: Further research is likely to have an important impact on our confidence in the estimate of effect and may change the estimate.
Low quality: Further research is very likely to have an important impact on our confidence in the estimate of effect and is likely to change the estimate.
Very low quality: We are very uncertain about the estimate.

1 There are high risk of bias.
2 Study includes relatively few patients and few events and thus has wide confidence intervals around the estimate of the effect.

舌三针 + 背俞穴埋线 + 基础治疗 VS 中风后假性球麻痹

Patient or population: patients with 中风后假性球麻痹
Intervention: 舌三针 + 背俞穴埋线 + 基础治疗 VS 常规针刺 + 基础治疗

Outcomes	Illustrative comparative risks* (95% CI)		Relative effect (95% CI)	No of Participants (studies)	Quality of the evidence (GRADE)	Comments
	Assumed risk	Corresponding risk				
	Control 舌三针 + 背俞穴埋线 + 基础治疗 VS 常规针刺 + 基础治疗					
	Study population					
临床总疗效 Follow – up: mean 3 months	767 per 1000	867 per 1000 (626 to 962)	OR 1.98 (0.51 to 7.63)	60 (1 study)	⊕○○○ very low[1,2]	
	Moderate					
	767 per 1000	867 per 1000 (627 to 962)				
洼田氏饮水试验评分 Follow – up: median 3 months		The mean 洼田氏饮水试验评分 in the intervention groups was 2.35 standard deviations higher (1.69 to 3.02 higher)		60 (1 study)	⊕○○○ very low[1,3]	SMD 2.35 (1.69 to 3.02)

* The basis for the assumed risk (e. g. the median control group risk across studies) is provided in footnotes. The corresponding risk (and its 95% confidence interval) is based on the assumed risk in the comparison group and the relative effect of the intervention (and its 95% CI).
CI: Confidence interval; OR: Odds ratio.

GRADE Working Group grades of evidence
High quality: Further research is very unlikely to change our confidence in the estimate of effect.
Moderate quality: Further research is likely to have an important impact on our confidence in the estimate of effect and may change the estimate.
Low quality: Further research is very likely to have an important impact on our confidence in the estimate of effect and is likely to change the estimate.
Very low quality: We are very uncertain about the estimate.

1 There are high risk of bias.
2 study include relatively few patients and few events and thus has wide confidence intervals around the estimate of the effect.
3 Study includes relatively few patients and few events.

电针＋基础治疗 VS 针刺＋基础治疗 for 中风后假性球麻痹

Patient or population: patients with 中风后假性球麻痹
Intervention: 电针＋基础治疗 VS 针刺＋基础治疗

Outcomes	Illustrative comparative risks* (95% CI)		Relative effect (95% CI)	No of Participants (studies)	Quality of the evidence (GRADE)	Comments
	Assumed risk	Corresponding risk				
	Control	电针＋基础治疗 VS 针刺＋基础治疗				
各项指标疗效评价 Follow－up: 3 months	Study population		OR 4.33 (1.2 to 15.61)	60 (1 study)	⊕⊕⊝⊝ very low[1,2]	
	600 per 1000	867 per 1000 (643 to 959)				
	Moderate					
	600 per 1000	867 per 1000 (643 to 959)				
各项指标评价积分	The mean 各项指标评价积分 in the intervention groups was 0.9 standard deviations lower (1.43 to 0.37 lower)			60 (1 study)	⊕⊕⊝⊝ low[1,3]	SMD －0.9 (－1.43 to －0.37)

* The basis for the assumed risk (e. g. the median control group risk across studies) is provided in footnotes. The corresponding risk (and its 95% confidence interval) is based on the assumed risk in the comparison group and the relative effect of the intervention (and its 95% CI).
CI: Confidence interval; OR: Odds ratio.

GRADE Working Group grades of evidence
High quality: Further research is very unlikely to change our confidence in the estimate of effect.
Moderate quality: Further research is likely to have an important impact on our confidence in the estimate of effect and may change the estimate.
Low quality: Further research is very likely to have an important impact on our confidence in the estimate of effect and is likely to change the estimate.
Very low quality: We are very uncertain about the estimate.

1 There are unclear risk of bias.
2 Study includes relatively few patients and few events and thus has wide confidence intervals around the estimate of the effect.
3 Study includes relatively few patients and few events.

舌下针 + 基础治疗 VS 基础治疗 for 中风后假性球麻痹

Patient or population: patients with 中风后假性球麻痹
Intervention: 舌下针 + 基础治疗 VS 基础治疗

Outcomes	Illustrative comparative risks* (95% CI)		Relative effect (95% CI)	No of Participants (studies)	Quality of the evidence (GRADE)	Comments
	Assumed risk	Corresponding risk				
	Control	舌下针 + 基础治疗 VS 基础治疗				
各项指标评价积分 Follow－up: 3 months		The mean 各项指标评价积分 in the intervention groups was 0.32 standard deviations lower (0.76 lower to 0.12 higher)		300 (1 study)	⊕⊕⊕⊖ very low[1,2,3]	SMD －0.32 (－0.76 to 0.12)
各项指标评价积分 － 总症状积分 Follow－up: 3 months		The mean 各项指标评价积分 － 总症状积分 in the intervention groups was 0.42 standard deviations higher (0.09 lower to 0.93 higher)		60 (1 study)	⊕⊕⊕⊖ low[1,3]	SMD 0.42 (－0.09 to 0.93)
各项指标评价积分 － 构音障碍 Follow－up: 3 months		The mean 各项指标评价积分 － 构音障碍 in the intervention groups was 0.84 standard deviations lower (1.37 to 0.31 lower)		60 (1 study)	⊕⊕⊕⊖ low[1,3]	SMD －0.84 (－1.37 to －0.31)
各项指标评价积分 － 吞咽障碍 Follow－up: 3 months		The mean 各项指标评价积分 － 吞咽障碍 in the intervention groups was 0.5 standard deviations lower (1.02 lower to 0.01 higher)		60 (1 study)	⊕⊕⊕⊖ low[1,3]	SMD －0.5 (－1.02 to 0.01)
各项指标评价积分 － 舌体运动 Follow－up: 3 months		The mean 各项指标评价积分 － 舌体运动 in the intervention groups was 0.63 standard deviations lower (1.15 to 0.11 lower)		60 (1 study)	⊕⊕⊕⊖ low[1,3]	SMD －0.63 (－1.15 to －0.11)
各项指标评价积分 － 情感状态 Follow－up: 3 months		The mean 各项指标评价积分 － 情感状态 in the intervention groups was 0.07 standard deviations lower (0.58 lower to 0.43 higher)		60 (1 study)	⊕⊕⊕⊖ low[1,3]	SMD －0.07 (－0.58 to 0.43)

* The basis for the assumed risk (e. g. the median control group risk across studies) is provided in footnotes. The corresponding risk (and its 95% confidence interval) is based on the assumed risk in the comparison group and the relative effect of the intervention (and its 95% CI).
CI: Confidence interval.

GRADE Working Group grades of evidence

High quality: Further research is very unlikely to change our confidence in the estimate of effect.
Moderate quality: Further research is likely to have an important impact on our confidence in the estimate of effect and may change the estimate.
Low quality: Further research is very likely to have an important impact on our confidence in the estimate of effect and is likely to change the estimate.
Very low quality: We are very uncertain about the estimate.

1 There are unclear risk of bias.
2 heterogeneity exists
3 Study includes relatively few patients and few events.

项针 + 基础治疗 VS 基础治疗 for 中风后假性球麻痹

Patient or population: patients with 中风后假性球麻痹
Intervention: 项针 + 基础治疗 VS 基础治疗

Outcomes	Illustrative comparative risks* (95% CI)		Relative effect (95% CI)	No of Participants (studies)	Quality of the evidence (GRADE)	Comments
	Assumed risk Control	Corresponding risk 项针 + 基础治疗 VS 基础治疗				
洼田饮水试验疗效评价 Follow – up: 3 months	Study population		OR 2.78 (1.06 to 7.34)	92 (1 study)	⊕⊕⊕⊝ low[1,2]	
	630 per 1000	826 per 1000 (644 to 926)				
	Moderate					
	630 per 1000	826 per 1000 (643 to 926)				
大西幸子吞咽功能疗效评价 Follow – up: 3 months	Study population		OR 6.66 (2.8 to 15.8)	256 (2 studies)	⊕⊕⊝⊝ very low[3,4]	
	727 per 1000	947 per 1000 (882 to 977)				
	Moderate					
	713 per 1000	943 per 1000 (874 to 975)				

续表

大西幸子言语功能疗效评价 Follow – up: 3 months	Study population		OR 4.58 (1. 79 to 11.71)	256 (2 studies)	⊕⊕⊝⊝ very low[3,4]
	531 per 1000	838 per 1000 (670 to 930)			
	Moderate				
	550 per 1000	848 per 1000 (686 to 935)			

* The basis for the assumed risk (e. g. the median control group risk across studies) is provided in footnotes. The corresponding risk (and its 95% confidence interval) is based on the assumed risk in the comparison group and the relative effect of the intervention (and its 95% CI).

CI: Confidence interval; OR: Odds ratio.

GRADE Working Group grades of evidence

High quality: Further research is very unlikely to change our confidence in the estimate of effect.

Moderate quality: Further research is likely to have an important impact on our confidence in the estimate of effect and may change the estimate.

Low quality: Further research is very likely to have an important impact on our confidence in the estimate of effect and is likely to change the estimate.

Very low quality: We are very uncertain about the estimate.

1 There are unclear risk of bias.

2 Study has wide confidence intervals around the estimate of the effect.

3 There are high risk of bias.

4 Studies have wide confidence intervals around the estimate of the effect.

颈项针 + 基础治疗 VS 舌三针 + 基础治疗 for 中风后假性球麻痹

Patient or population: patients with 中风后假性球麻痹
Intervention: 颈项针 + 基础治疗 VS 舌三针 + 基础治疗

Outcomes	Illustrative comparative risks * (95% CI)		Relative effect (95% CI)	No of Participants (studies)	Quality of the evidence (GRADE)	Comments
	Assumed risk Control 颈项针 + 基础治疗 VS 舌三针 + 基础治疗	Corresponding risk 颈项针 + 基础治疗 VS 舌三针 + 基础治疗				
中医疗效评价 Follow – up: 3 months	Study population		OR 2.02 (0.69 to 5.87)	120 (1 study)	⊕⊕⊝⊝ very low[1,2]	
	817 per 1000	900 per 1000 (755 to 963)				
	Moderate					
	817 per 1000	900 per 1000 (755 to 963)				
中医病症状体征积分 Follow – up: 3 months	The mean 中医病症状体征积分 in the intervention groups was 0.36 standard deviations higher (0 to 0.72 higher)			120 (1 study)	⊕⊕⊕⊝ low[1,2]	SMD 0.36 (0 to 0.72)

* The basis for the assumed risk (e. g. the median control group risk across studies) is provided in footnotes. The corresponding risk (and its 95% confidence interval) is based on the assumed risk in the comparison group and the relative effect of the intervention (and its 95% CI).

CI: Confidence interval; OR: Odds ratio.

GRADE Working Group grades of evidence
High quality: Further research is very unlikely to change our confidence in the estimate of effect.
Moderate quality: Further research is likely to have an important impact on our confidence in the estimate of effect and may change the estimate.
Low quality: Further research is very likely to have an important impact on our confidence in the estimate of effect and is likely to change the estimate.
Very low quality: We are very uncertain about the estimate.

1 There are high risk of bias.
2 Study has wide confidence intervals around the estimate of the effect.

醒脑开药针刺法＋基础治疗 VS 常规针刺法＋基础治疗 for 中风后假性球麻痹

Patient or population: patients with 中风后假性球麻痹
Intervention: 醒脑开药针刺法＋基础治疗 VS 常规针刺法＋基础治疗

Outcomes	Illustrative comparative risks* (95% CI)		Relative effect (95% CI)	No of Participants (studies)	Quality of the evidence (GRADE)	Comments
	Assumed risk	Corresponding risk				
	Control 醒脑开药针刺法＋基础治疗 VS 常规针刺法＋基础治疗					
	Study population					
中医病疗效评价 Follow－up: 3 months	819 per 1000	954 per 1000 (868 to 985)	OR 4.56 (1.45 to 14.4)	170 (2 studies)	⊕⊕⊖⊖ low[1,2]	
	Moderate					
	819 per 1000	954 per 1000 (868 to 985)				

* The basis for the assumed risk (e.g. the median control group risk across studies) is provided in footnotes. The corresponding risk (and its 95% confidence interval) is based on the assumed risk in the comparison group and the relative effect of the intervention (and its 95% CI).
CI: Confidence interval; OR: Odds ratio.

GRADE Working Group grades of evidence
High quality: Further research is very unlikely to change our confidence in the estimate of effect.
Moderate quality: Further research is likely to have an important impact on our confidence in the estimate of effect and may change the estimate.
Low quality: Further research is very likely to have an important impact on our confidence in the estimate of effect and is likely to change the estimate.
Very low quality: We are very uncertain about the estimate.

1 There are unclear risk of bias.
2 studies has wide confidence intervals around the estimate of the effect.

醒脑开窍针法＋基础治疗 VS 基础治疗 for 中风后假性球麻痹

Patient or population: patients with 中风后假性球麻痹
Intervention: 醒脑开窍针法＋基础治疗 VS 基础治疗

Outcomes	Illustrative comparative risks * (95% CI)		Relative effect (95% CI)	No of Participants (studies)	Quality of the evidence (GRADE)	Comments
	Assumed risk	Corresponding risk				
	Control	醒脑开窍针法＋基础治疗 VS 基础治疗				
	Study population					
吞咽功能疗效评价 Follow－up: 3 months	596 per 1000	941 per 1000 (835 to 981)	OR 10.84 (3.42 to 34.3)	120 (1 study)	⊕⊕⊝⊝ very low[1,2]	
	Moderate					
	596 per 1000	941 per 1000 (835 to 981)				
洼田饮水试验评分 Follow－up: 3 months	The mean 洼田饮水试验评分 in the intervention groups was 0.87 standard deviations higher (0.49 to 1.25 higher)			120 (1 study)	⊕⊕⊝⊝ low[1,2]	SMD 0.87 (0.49 to 1.25)

* The basis for the assumed risk (e.g. the median control group risk across studies) is provided in footnotes. The corresponding risk (and its 95% confidence interval) is based on the assumed risk in the comparison group and the relative effect of the intervention (and its 95% CI).

CI: Confidence interval; OR: Odds ratio.

GRADE Working Group grades of evidence
High quality: Further research is very unlikely to change our confidence in the estimate of effect.
Moderate quality: Further research is likely to have an important impact on our confidence in the estimate of effect and may change the estimate.
Low quality: Further research is very likely to have an important impact on our confidence in the estimate of effect and is likely to change the estimate.
Very low quality: We are very uncertain about the estimate.

1 There are high risk of bias.
2 Study has wide confidence intervals around the estimate of the effect.

舌咽针 + 基础疗法 VS 基础疗法 for 中风后假性球麻痹

Patient or population: patients with 中风后假性球麻痹
Intervention: 舌咽针 + 基础疗法 VS 基础疗法

Outcomes	Illustrative comparative risks* (95% CI)		Relative effect (95% CI)	No of Participants (studies)	Quality of the evidence (GRADE)	Comments
	Assumed risk Control	Corresponding risk 舌咽针 + 基础疗法 VS 基础疗法				
临床症状疗效评价 Follow-up: 3 months	Study population		OR 4.46 (0.47 to 42.51)	60 (1 study)	⊕⊖⊖⊖ very low[1,2]	
	867 per 1000	967 per 1000 (753 to 996)				
	Moderate					
	867 per 1000	967 per 1000 (754 to 996)				
进田饮水试验疗效评价 Follow-up: 3 months	Study population		OR 3.27 (0.77 to 13.83)	60 (1 study)	⊕⊖⊖⊖ very low[1,2]	
	733 per 1000	900 per 1000 (679 to 974)				
	Moderate					
	733 per 1000	900 per 1000 (679 to 974)				

* The basis for the assumed risk (e. g. the median control group risk across studies) is provided in footnotes. The corresponding risk (and its 95% confidence interval) is based on the assumed risk in the comparison group and the relative effect of the intervention (and its 95% CI).

CI: Confidence interval; OR: Odds ratio.

GRADE Working Group grades of evidence

High quality: Further research is very unlikely to change our confidence in the estimate of effect.

Moderate quality: Further research is likely to have an important impact on our confidence in the estimate of effect and may change the estimate.

Low quality: Further research is very likely to have an important impact on our confidence in the estimate of effect and is likely to change the estimate.

Very low quality: We are very uncertain about the estimate.

1 There are unclear risk of bias.

2 Study includes relatively few patients and few events and thus has wide confidence intervals around the estimate of the effect.

舌咽针 + 基础治疗 VS 常规针刺 + 基础治疗 for 中风后假性球麻痹

Patient or population: patients with 中风后假性球麻痹
Intervention: 舌咽针 + 基础治疗 VS 常规针刺 + 基础治疗

Outcomes	Illustrative comparative risks* (95% CI)		Relative effect (95% CI)	No of Participants (studies)	Quality of the evidence (GRADE)	Comments
	Assumed risk Control	Corresponding risk 舌咽针 + 基础治疗 VS 常规针刺 + 基础治疗				
	Study population					
洼田饮水试验疗效评价 Follow-up: 3 months	717 per 1000	920 per 1000 (796 to 971)	OR 4.53 (1.54 to 13.31)	121 (2 studies)	⊕⊝⊝⊝ very low[1,2]	
	Moderate					
	717 per 1000	920 per 1000 (796 to 971)				

* The basis for the assumed risk (e. g. the median control group risk across studies) is provided in footnotes. The corresponding risk (and its 95% confidence interval) is based on the assumed risk in the comparison group and the relative effect of the intervention (and its 95% CI).

CI: Confidence interval; OR: Odds ratio.

GRADE Working Group grades of evidence
High quality: Further research is very unlikely to change our confidence in the estimate of effect.
Moderate quality: Further research is likely to have an important impact on our confidence in the estimate of effect and may change the estimate.
Low quality: Further research is very likely to have an important impact on our confidence in the estimate of effect and is likely to change the estimate.
Very low quality: We are very uncertain about the estimate.

1 There are unclear risk of bias.
2 Studies include relatively few patients and few events and thus have wide confidence intervals around the estimate of the effect.

穴位注射 + 基础治疗 VS 基础治疗 for 中风后假性球麻痹

Patient or population: patients with 中风后假性球麻痹
Intervention: 穴位注射 + 基础治疗 VS 基础治疗

Outcomes	Illustrative comparative risks * (95% CI)		Relative effect (95% CI)	No of Participants (studies)	Quality of the evidence (GRADE)	Comments
	Assumed risk	Corresponding risk				
	Control	穴位注射 + 基础治疗 VS 基础治疗				
	Study population					
临床症状疗效评价	735 per 1000	964 per 1000 (921 to 984)	OR 9.7 (4.22 to 22.27)	367 (2 studies)	⊕⊝⊝⊝ very low[1,2]	
Follow – up: 3 months	Moderate					
	740 per 1000	965 per 1000 (923 to 984)				

* The basis for the assumed risk (e.g. the median control group risk across studies) is provided in footnotes. The corresponding risk (and its 95% confidence interval) is based on the assumed risk in the comparison group and the relative effect of the intervention (and its 95% CI).
CI: Confidence interval; OR: Odds ratio.

GRADE Working Group grades of evidence
High quality: Further research is very unlikely to change our confidence in the estimate of effect.
Moderate quality: Further research is likely to have an important impact on our confidence in the estimate of effect and may change the estimate.
Low quality: Further research is very likely to have an important impact on our confidence in the estimate of effect and is likely to change the estimate.
Very low quality: We are very uncertain about the estimate.

1 There are high risk of bias.
2 studies have wide confidence intervals around the estimate of the effect.

穴位注射＋基础治疗 VS 常规针刺＋基础治疗 for 中风后假性球麻痹

Patient or population: patients with 中风后假性球麻痹

Intervention: 穴位注射＋基础治疗 VS 常规针刺＋基础治疗

Outcomes	Illustrative comparative risks* (95% CI)		Relative effect (95% CI)	No of Participants (studies)	Quality of the evidence (GRADE)	Comments
	Assumed risk	Corresponding risk				
	Control	穴位注射＋基础治疗 VS 常规针刺＋基础治疗				
	Study population					
淮田饮水试验疗效评价	700 per 1000	933 per 1000 (732 to 986)	OR 6 (1.17 to 30.72)	60 (1 study)	⊕⊝⊝⊝ very low[1,2,3]	
Follow－up: 3 months	Moderate					
	700 per 1000	933 per 1000 (732 to 986)				

* The basis for the assumed risk (e. g. the median control group risk across studies) is provided in footnotes. The corresponding risk (and its 95% confidence interval) is based on the assumed risk in the comparison group and the relative effect of the intervention (and its 95% CI).

CI: Confidence interval; OR: Odds ratio.

GRADE Working Group grades of evidence

High quality: Further research is very unlikely to change our confidence in the estimate of effect.

Moderate quality: Further research is likely to have an important impact on our confidence in the estimate of effect and may change the estimate.

Low quality: Further research is very likely to have an important impact on our confidence in the estimate of effect and is likely to change the estimate.

Very low quality: We are very uncertain about the estimate.

1 There are high risk of bias.

2 No explanation was provided.

3 Study includes relatively few patients and few events and thus has wide confidence intervals around the estimate of the effect.

耳针 + 常规针刺 + 基础疗法 VS 常规针刺 + 基础疗法 for 中风后假性球麻痹

Patient or population: patients with 中风后假性球麻痹
Intervention: 耳针 + 常规针刺 + 基础疗法 VS 常规针刺 + 基础疗法

Outcomes	Illustrative comparative risks * (95% CI)		Relative effect (95% CI)	No of Participants (studies)	Quality of the evidence (GRADE)	Comments
	Assumed risk	Corresponding risk				
	Control	耳针 + 常规针刺 + 基础疗法 VS 常规针刺 + 基础疗法				
	Study population					
洼田饮水试验疗效评价 Follow – up: 3 months	643 per 1000	786 per 1000 (406 to 952)	OR 2. 04 (0. 38 to 10. 94)	28 (1 study)	⊕○○○ very low[1,2]	
	Moderate					
	643 per 1000	786 per 1000 (406 to 952)				
洼田饮水试验评分 Follow – up: 3 months		The mean 洼田饮水试验评分 in the intervention groups was 2.85 standard deviations higher (1. 75 to 3. 94 higher)		28 (1 study)	⊕○○○ very low[1,2]	SMD 2. 85 (1. 75 to 3. 94)

* The basis for the assumed risk (e. g. the median control group risk across studies) is provided in footnotes. The corresponding risk (and its 95% confidence interval) is based on the assumed risk in the comparison group and the relative effect of the intervention (and its 95% CI).
CI: Confidence interval; OR: Odds ratio.

GRADE Working Group grades of evidence
High quality: Further research is very unlikely to change our confidence in the estimate of effect.
Moderate quality: Further research is likely to have an important impact on our confidence in the estimate of effect and may change the estimate.
Low quality: Further research is very likely to have an important impact on our confidence in the estimate of effect and is likely to change the estimate.
Very low quality: We are very uncertain about the estimate.

1 There are high risk of bias.
2 Study includes relatively few patients and few events and thus has wide confidence intervals around the estimate of the effect.

康复训练 + 针刺 + 基础治疗 VS 针刺 + 基础治疗 for 中风后假性球麻痹

Patient or population: patients with 中风后假性球麻痹
Intervention: 康复训练 + 针刺 + 基础治疗 VS 针刺 + 基础治疗

Outcomes	Illustrative comparative risks* (95% CI)		Relative effect (95% CI)	No of Participants (studies)	Quality of the evidence (GRADE)	Comments
	Assumed risk Control	Corresponding risk 康复训练 + 针刺 + 基础治疗 VS 针刺 + 基础治疗				
构音障碍疗效评价 Follow – up: 3 months	Study population		OR 3.67 (1.41 to 9.51)	84 (1 study)	⊕⊝⊝⊝ very low[1,2]	
	500 per 1000	786 per 1000 (585 to 905)				
	Moderate					
	500 per 1000	786 per 1000 (585 to 905)				
洼田饮水试验评分 Follow – up: 3 months	The mean 洼田饮水试验评分 in the intervention groups was 0.19 standard deviations higher (0.21 lower to 0.59 higher)			96 (1 study)	⊕⊕⊝⊝ low[1,2]	SMD 0.19 (−0.21 to 0.59)

* The basis for the assumed risk (e. g. the median control group risk across studies) is provided in footnotes. The corresponding risk (and its 95% confidence interval) is based on the assumed risk in the comparison group and the relative effect of the intervention (and its 95% CI).
CI: Confidence interval; OR: Odds ratio.

GRADE Working Group grades of evidence
High quality: Further research is very unlikely to change our confidence in the estimate of effect.
Moderate quality: Further research is likely to have an important impact on our confidence in the estimate of effect and may change the estimate.
Low quality: Further research is very likely to have an important impact on our confidence in the estimate of effect and is likely to change the estimate.
Very low quality: We are very uncertain about the estimate.

1 There are high risk of bias.
2 Study has wide confidence intervals around the estimate of the effect.

靳三针＋基础治疗 VS 常规针刺＋基础治疗 for 中风后假性球麻痹

Patient or population: patients with 中风后假性球麻痹
Intervention: 靳三针＋基础治疗 VS 常规针刺＋基础治疗

Outcomes	Illustrative comparative risks* (95% CI)		Relative effect (95% CI)	No of Participants (studies)	Quality of the evidence (GRADE)	Comments
	Assumed risk Control	Corresponding risk 靳三针＋基础治疗 VS 常规针刺＋基础治疗				
症状体征疗效评价 Follow-up: 3 months	Study population		OR 1 (0.27 to 3.76)	80 (1 study)	⊕◯◯◯ very low [1,2]	
	875 per 1000	875 per 1000 (654 to 963)				
	Moderate					
	875 per 1000	875 per 1000 (654 to 963)				
症状体征积分评价 Follow-up: 3 months		The mean 症状体征积分评价 in the intervention groups was 0.76 standard deviations higher (0.31 to 1.22 higher)		80 (1 study)	⊕◯◯◯ very low [1,3]	SMD 0.76 (0.31 to 1.22)

* The basis for the assumed risk (e. g. the median control group risk across studies) is provided in footnotes. The corresponding risk (and its 95% confidence interval) is based on the assumed risk in the comparison group and the relative effect of the intervention (and its 95% CI).
CI: Confidence interval; OR: Odds ratio.

GRADE Working Group grades of evidence
High quality: Further research is very unlikely to change our confidence in the estimate of effect.
Moderate quality: Further research is likely to have an important impact on our confidence in the estimate of effect and may change the estimate.
Low quality: Further research is very likely to have an important impact on our confidence in the estimate of effect and is likely to change the estimate.
Very low quality: We are very uncertain about the estimate.

1 There are high risk of bias.
2 Study includes relatively few patients and few events and thus has wide confidence intervals around the estimate of the effect.
3 Study includes relatively few patients and few events.

耳三针 + 基础治疗 VS 基础治疗 for 中风后假性球麻痹

Patient or population: patients with 中风后假性球麻痹
Intervention: 耳三针 + 基础治疗 VS 基础治疗

Outcomes	Illustrative comparative risks* (95% CI)		Relative effect (95% CI)	No of Participants (studies)	Quality of the evidence (GRADE)	Comments
	Assumed risk	Corresponding risk				
	Control	耳三针 + 基础治疗 VS 基础治疗				
洼田饮水试验评分 Follow-up: 3 months		The mean 洼田饮水试验评分 in the intervention groups was 0.63 standard deviations higher (0.18 to 1.08 higher)		80 (1 study)	⊕⊝⊝⊝ very low[1,2]	SMD 0.63 (0.18 to 1.08)
藤岛一郎吞咽障碍评分 Follow-up: 3 months		The mean 藤岛一郎吞咽障碍评分 in the intervention groups was 0.43 standard deviations lower (0.88 lower to 0.01 higher)		80 (1 study)	⊕⊝⊝⊝ very low[1,2]	SMD -0.43 (-0.88 to 0.01)

* The basis for the assumed risk (e. g. the median control group risk across studies) is provided in footnotes. The corresponding risk (and its 95% confidence interval) is based on the assumed risk in the comparison group and the relative effect of the intervention (and its 95% CI).

CI: Confidence interval.

GRADE Working Group grades of evidence
High quality: Further research is very unlikely to change our confidence in the estimate of effect.
Moderate quality: Further research is likely to have an important impact on our confidence in the estimate of effect and may change the estimate.
Low quality: Further research is very likely to have an important impact on our confidence in the estimate of effect and is likely to change the estimate.
Very low quality: We are very uncertain about the estimate.

1 There are high risk of bias.
2 Study includes relatively few patients and few events.

深刺人迎穴 + 常规针刺 + 基础治疗 VS 常规针刺 + 基础治疗 for 中风后假性球麻痹

Patient or population: patients with 中风后假性球麻痹
Intervention: 深刺人迎穴 + 常规针刺 + 基础治疗 VS 常规针刺 + 基础治疗

Outcomes	Illustrative comparative risks* (95% CI)		Relative effect (95% CI)	No of Participants (studies)	Quality of the evidence (GRADE)	Comments
	Assumed risk	Corresponding risk				
	Control 深刺人迎穴 + 常规针刺 + 基础治疗 VS 常规针刺 + 基础治疗					
洼田饮水试验疗效评价 Follow – up: 3 months	Study population		OR 4.67 (1.45 to 15.05)	120 (1 study)	⊕⊕⊕⊝ low[1,2]	
	750 per 1000	933 per 1000 (813 to 978)				
	Moderate					
	750 per 1000	933 per 1000 (813 to 978)				
洼田饮水试验评分 Follow – up: 3 months		The mean 洼田饮水试验评分 in the intervention groups was 2.41 standard deviations higher (1.93 to 2.88 higher)		120 (1 study)	⊕⊕⊕⊝ low[1,2]	SMD 2.41 (1.93 to 2.88)

* The basis for the assumed risk (e. g. the median control group risk across studies) is provided in footnotes. The corresponding risk (and its 95% confidence interval) is based on the assumed risk in the comparison group and the relative effect of the intervention (and its 95% CI).
CI: Confidence interval; OR: Odds ratio.

GRADE Working Group grades of evidence
High quality: Further research is very unlikely to change our confidence in the estimate of effect.
Moderate quality: Further research is likely to have an important impact on our confidence in the estimate of effect and may change the estimate.
Low quality: Further research is very likely to have an important impact on our confidence in the estimate of effect and is likely to change the estimate.
Very low quality: We are very uncertain about the estimate.

1 There are unclear risk of bias.
2 Study has wide confidence intervals around the estimate of the effect.

6 本《指南》推荐方案的形成过程

6.1 确定《指南》推荐方案框架

中风一病涉及症状很多，很难在一个《指南》里将所有的内容同时囊括，因此，对于初次编写针灸指南来讲，选择一个合适的病种是很关键的。假性球麻痹属于中风病中的一个症候，具有明确的诊断，症状单一，便于进行临床疗效评价，而且针灸治疗具有明显的优势，因此，适于作为范例进行《指南》编写。题目内容的缩小，使针灸治疗目的更加具体化，更符合临床实际。

6.2 文献的检索与筛选

中英文数据库的检索，按照一定的检索策略，检索目标文献，按照文献纳入和排除标准对文献进行筛选，并通过电话或邮件联系作者，确定研究的真实性，了解相关详细信息。

古代文献、近现代专家专著或经验证据的检索，以电子检索为主，结合手工检索，务必搜集全所有制定专著文献。

6.3 决定结局指标重要程度分级

项目专家组成员根据所有结局对患者的重要程度，区分关键结局和重要但非关键结局。采用 9 级分级判断结局的重要程度。7～9 级为决策必须考虑的关键重要结局；4～6 级代表重要但非关键结局；1～3 级为不太重要的结局。

6.4 文献质量评估

提取纳入 RCT 的相关数据，利用 Cochrane Handbook 5.0 推荐的"偏倚风险评估"工具对纳入研究进行方法学质量评价；然后采用 Cochrane Review Manager 软件对不同针灸相关疗法治疗 AR 的有效性进行 Meta 分析；最后应用 GRADE 系统推荐分级方法对系统评价结果进行证据质量评估。GRADE 软件将证据质量分为高、中、低、极低 4 级，本标准建议采用字母描述法（ABCD 四个级别）。

6.5 推荐意见的形成

根据文献证据质量，在充分考虑到干预措施的利弊关系、患者意愿价值观、费用等情况下，通过专家问卷或会议的形式，形成不同具体针灸疗法的推荐。

在决定推荐的具体针灸疗法后，按照不同目标人群、疾病的不同阶段、不同的治疗原则与针灸方法、疗效评价指标等因素，将现代文献、古代文献及名医家经验证据进行归类，再合并形成证据群。在充分考虑到针灸疗法的安全性、实用性及可推广性后，通过专家共识的方法，形成初步推荐意见。

推荐强度反映了对一项干预措施是否利大于弊的确定程度。推荐方案的强度分为强推荐、弱推荐两个层次。项目组用"强推荐"表示确信相关的干预措施利大于弊。用"弱推荐"表示干预措施有可能利大于弊，但把握不大。

决定推荐强度的关键因素有四个：第一个关键因素是在充分权衡不同治疗方案利弊基础上的利弊平衡。第二个关键因素是证据质量。第三个关键因素是患者价值观和意愿的不确定或多变性。第四个关键因素是费用。成本比其他因素更易受时间、地理区域影响而变化。

6.6 推荐方案初稿形成

由起草组综合各治疗方案及其推荐意见，形成《指南》推荐方案初稿。

6.7 修订推荐方案

项目组组织推荐方案的修订及完善工作。采用会议、函审等多种形式，进行多轮次专家咨询，根据《指南》的适用范围及临床实际使用情况，对《指南》的推荐方案进行修订和完善。

6.8 确定推荐方案终稿

项目组召开扩大的项目组专家委员会会议，遵循罗伯特会议规则，以会审的形式确定推荐方案终稿。

7 本《指南》推荐方案征求意见稿

7.1 针灸治疗中风后假性球麻痹的原则及特点

7.1.1 治疗总则

针灸治疗中风后假性球麻痹的总原则为辨症施治。

7.1.2 选穴处方特点

中风后假性球麻痹以吞咽困难和构音障碍为主要临床表现，针灸治疗中风后假性球麻痹建议以对症选穴为主，结合循经远端选穴和/或辨证选穴。

对症选穴：通常选取项部和颈部的穴位。根据本病病位在脑，累及舌咽的特点，颈部常用腧穴有廉泉、夹廉泉、人迎等，项部常用腧穴有风池、风府、哑门、完骨等。病情轻者，可以项部腧穴为主；病情重者，建议颈、项部腧穴同用。具体见附图1至附图3[7]。

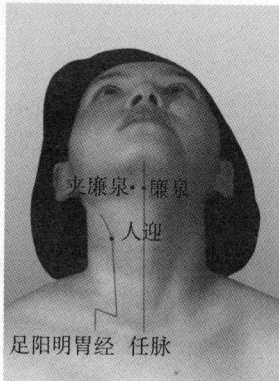

附图1 头颈部经络
腧穴示意图（正面）

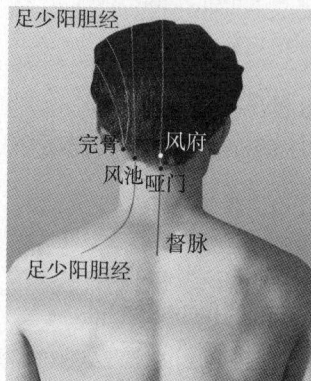

附图2 头项部经络
腧穴示意图（背面）

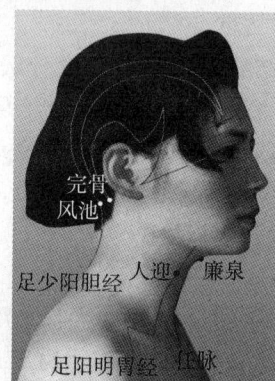

附图3 头颈部经络
腧穴示意图（右侧位）

循经远端取穴：循行至咽喉部的经脉有足少阴肾经、足阳明胃经、足厥阴肝经、手太阴肺经、阴阳跷脉等，常用的腧穴如列缺、照海、通里、丰隆、三阴交、内关等穴。

辨证取穴：根据不同的辨证分型[6]，选取相应的腧穴。如肝阳上亢配太冲，风痰阻络配丰隆，瘀血阻窍配足三里、三阴交，肾精亏虚配太溪、太冲等。

针灸治疗中风后假性球麻痹要以对症选穴为主，重视辨症选穴与辨证选穴相结合，近部选穴与远端选穴相结合。

7.1.3 辨证选穴处方特点

中风后假性球麻痹是由于双侧上运动神经元损伤所造成的，病因中最常见的是高血压和动脉硬化性脑血管病，尤其是反复发作的双侧脑血管病，因此临床上常见偏侧肢体功能活动障碍、吞咽困难和构音障碍、情感障碍、认知障碍等。

中风后假性球麻痹首先要重点治疗主要症状，同时不能忽视并发症的针灸治疗。中风后假性球麻痹伴有偏瘫的患者在针对主症治疗的同时，可以配伍肩髃、曲池、外关、合谷、后溪、环跳、足三里、阳陵泉、悬钟等；强哭强笑者，配伍百会、印堂、人中等；中枢性尿失禁，配伍四神聪、百会。

7.1.4 疗程

大多数文献报道每日治疗1次，5～10次为1疗程，疗程间休息1～2天。

7.1.5 针灸干预时机

目前对针灸治疗中风后假性球麻痹的干预时机尚没有明确结论，但从临床研究文献看，治疗时间最早者为发病1日内[8]，并无不良反应。一般认为，中风后假性球麻痹采用针刺干预的时间越早越好[45]，发病20天内针刺，其疗效优于20天后，但发病10天内与11～20天内开始治疗相比，其疗效差异不明显[46]，此结论还有待进一步临床验证。

7.2 推荐方案

7.2.1 穴组方案推荐

7.2.1.1 对症选穴

`颈部取穴`

取穴：廉泉、夹廉泉、人迎、扶突。

针刺方法：人迎，位于喉结尖旁开1.5寸，颈总动脉内侧缘，直刺1~1.5寸，局部有窒息样针感。廉泉，施以合谷刺法，先向舌根方向刺入1.5~1.8寸，再向左右各刺入1.5~1.8寸，以局部得气为宜。夹廉泉，位于廉泉同一水平旁开0.5寸，针尖向舌根方向，进针1.2~1.5寸，局部有酸胀感即可。扶突，向喉头方向斜刺，深约1寸，以针感向喉头放射为佳。以上4穴均得气后施以平补平泻手法。

电针操作：双侧夹廉泉可以接电针治疗仪，采用疏密波，以病人耐受为度。

穴位注射：廉泉穴位注射，令患者仰卧，用5mL注射器抽取药液（临床常用B族维生素），7号长针头针尖朝向舌根方向刺入2寸左右，舌体有针感后推入药液，每穴1mL。

颈部取穴横断面解剖图见附图4、附图5[7]。

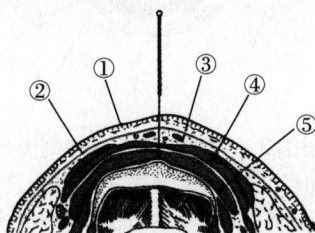

附图4 廉泉穴横断面图示
①皮肤；②皮下组织；③针在左、右二腹肌前腹之间通过；④下颌舌骨肌；⑤颏舌骨肌

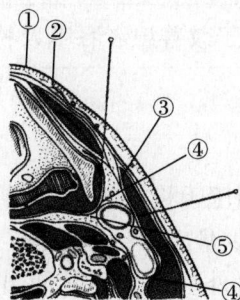

附图5 人迎穴横断面图示
①皮肤；②皮下组织和颈阔肌；③颈固有筋膜浅层及胸锁乳突肌；④颈固有筋膜深层；⑤咽缩肌

注意事项：针刺颈项部穴位要充分注意针刺的深度和方向。针刺人迎时，应避开颈总动脉。

『推荐』

> 廉泉、夹廉泉、人迎、扶突主要用于改善患者吞咽及构音功能。[CRADE 1C]

`项部取穴`

取穴：风府、风池、哑门、百劳。

针刺方法：风府，针尖朝向喉结方向，进针1~1.2寸。风池，针尖稍向内下方，刺入1~1.5寸。哑门，针尖向下颌方向缓慢刺入0.5~1寸。百劳，直刺1.2寸。诸穴以局部有酸胀感为宜。

电针操作：双侧风池可以接电针治疗仪，采用疏密波，以病人耐受为度。

穴位注射：风池、哑门穴位注射，用5mL注射器抽取药液（临床常用B族维生素），以7号长针头针刺，进针得气后每穴注射药液1mL。

项部取穴横断面解剖见附图6、附图7[7]。

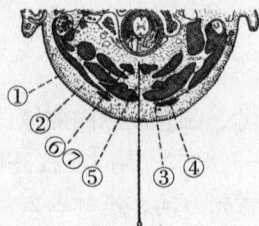

附图6　风府穴横断面解剖图示
①皮肤；②皮下组织；③斜方肌腱；④头半棘肌；⑤项韧带；⑥头后小直肌；⑦头后大直肌

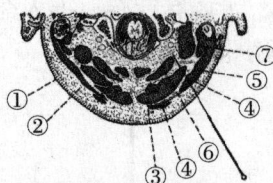

附图7　风池穴横断面解剖图示
①皮肤；②皮下组织；③斜方肌和胸锁乳突肌之间通过；④头夹肌；
⑤头半棘肌；⑥针的内侧为头后大直肌；⑦针的外侧为头上斜肌

注意事项：风府、哑门不可向上斜刺过深，以免伤及深部延髓。

『推荐』

> 风府、风池、哑门、百劳穴主要用于改善患者吞咽及构音功能。[CRADE 1C]

其他部位取穴

取穴：咽后壁、金津、玉液。

操作方法：咽后壁，令患者张口，用压舌板将舌体向后下方推压，以长度75～100mm的芒针点刺悬雍垂两侧之咽后壁，每侧3～5针，少量出血，不留针。

金津、玉液，让患者自然将舌伸出口外（如舌不能伸出者，可由医者垫纱布固定舌体于口外），常规消毒二穴，用毫针点刺少量出血，不留针。

注意事项：点刺后令患者保持低头位，避免血液回流气管引发呼吸道堵塞。

『推荐』

> 咽后壁和金津、玉液穴对构音功能有明显的改善作用。[CRADE 2B]

7.2.1.2　循经远端取穴

取穴：列缺与照海，通里与内关，丰隆与三阴交，合谷与太冲。

针刺方法：以上腧穴常规针刺，平补平泻。

电针操作：丰隆与三阴交、合谷与太冲可以接电针治疗仪，采用疏密波，以病人耐受为度。

『推荐』

> 循经远端取穴是针灸处方的重要组成部分，尤其是循经远端对穴的配伍应用，可以增进穴位间的相互协调作用，增强疗效。[CRADE 2B]

7.2.1.3 辨证取穴

取穴：肝阳上亢型加太冲、太溪，风痰阻络配丰隆、中脘，瘀血阻窍配足三里、三阴交，肾精亏虚配太溪、肾俞。

针刺操作方法：根据"虚则补之，实则泻之"的原则，太冲、丰隆、三阴交施提插捻转泻法，足三里、太溪施提插捻转补法。

电针操作：以上穴位选取一组或两组，接通电针治疗仪，采用疏密波，以病人耐受为度。

『推荐』

> 辨证取穴对于治病求本、巩固临床疗效有重要的意义。[CRADE 2D]

7.2.2 处方方案推荐

根据患者情况，选取一种或两种以上取穴方案，构成针灸处方。

7.2.2.1 体针疗法

临床上治疗中风后假性球麻痹往往病症兼顾。在治疗原发病的同时，临床常用对症选穴方案。

取穴：风府、百劳、人迎、廉泉、夹廉泉。

针刺方法：具体针刺方法可见本章节7.2.1.1。

电针疗法：针刺得气后，夹廉泉接通电针治疗仪，采用疏密波，以患者耐受为度。

疗程：每日治疗1次，15天为1个疗程。

注意事项：高血压患者，针刺人迎时针感不宜过强。

『推荐』

> 本方案适用于中风各期的一般假性球麻痹患者。[CRADE 1B]

7.2.2.2 项针疗法

项针疗法是黑龙江中医药大学附属第一医院高维滨、唐强等创立的一种特殊针灸疗法，用于治疗假性球麻痹疗效显著。自1996年至今已有多年的临床应用经验，目前在东北地区、全国部分地区的医院应用。

取穴：风池、翳明、治呛（甲状软骨上切迹上缘与舌骨下缘之间，直刺1寸以内），供血（风池穴直下1.5寸，向内侧直刺1寸）、吞咽（喉结与舌骨体中点，旁开0.5寸，向内侧稍斜刺0.3寸）、发音（甲状软骨与环状软骨的中点，旁开0.2寸，直刺0.3寸）、治反流（发音穴外0.5寸，向内侧斜刺0.3寸）、廉泉、外金津、玉液。

针刺方法：风池、翳明、供血，针尖稍向内下方，刺入1~1.5寸。廉泉、外金津、玉液，向舌根刺入1.2~1.5寸。治呛、吞咽直刺0.3寸。发音、治反流穴直刺0.2寸。

电针：吞咽障碍明显者，治呛接电针；构音障碍明显者，发音穴接电针。电针治疗仪采用疏密波，以患者耐受为度。

疗程：每日上、下午各治疗1次。5天为1个疗程，疗程间休息1天。

『推荐』

> 本方案适用于中风各期的一般假性球麻痹患者。[CRADE 2C]

7.2.2.3 醒脑开窍法

此疗法为天津中医药大学附属第一医院石学敏院士于1972年开创，经过30多年的临床反复实践应用，证实有较好的临床疗效。目前国内除天津地区外，许多省、市、县级医院都有应用的报道。

取穴：风池、翳风或完骨、三阴交、内关、水沟。

针刺方法：风池、翳风或完骨穴，均针向结喉，震颤徐入2.5寸，小幅度、高频率捻转1分钟，以咽喉部麻胀感为宜。三阴交，直刺1~1.5寸，行提插补法1分钟。水沟，行雀啄刺，使眼球湿润或流泪为度。内关，行提插捻转泻法1分钟。

疗程：首次治疗先刺水沟、内关，以后可2~3天针刺1次；风池、翳风或完骨、三阴交每日1次。10次为1个疗程，疗程间休息2天。

『推荐』

> 本方案适用于中风各期的一般假性球麻痹患者。[CRADE 1C]

7.2.2.4 头体针结合疗法

此疗法是头针与体针结合，兼具头、体针两种疗法的综合疗效，临床报道疗效较好。

头针取穴：顶中线、顶颞前斜线、顶颞后斜线、顶旁1线、顶旁2线。

体针取穴：风池、翳风、廉泉、金津、玉液。

针刺方法：①头针操作：沿头皮呈15°角斜刺至帽状腱膜下，进针1~1.5寸，采用提插手法，进针时幅度小，行针时提插幅度要大。每穴行针时间约30秒，可两针同时操作。边行针边嘱患者尽量活动相应肢体，得气后留针，连接电针治疗仪，断续波，低频，以患者耐受为度，留针30分钟，每日2次，上午针患侧，下午针健侧。②体针操作：取风池、翳风（针尖对准喉结方向进针2.5寸）、廉泉、金津、玉液，针刺得气后，采用平补平泻手法，留针30分钟。采用相同的腧穴及操作，上、下午各治疗1次。

疗程：15天为1个疗程，疗程间休息2天。

注意事项：脑出血开颅术后患者慎用本法。

『推荐』

> 本方案适用于中风恢复期、后遗症期以半身不遂、假性球麻痹为主症者。[CRADE 1C]

7.2.2.5 放血疗法

此疗法是针灸治疗中风后假性球麻痹的常用方法之一，临床报道疗效较好。

取穴：咽后壁、翳风、内关。

针刺方法：令患者张口，用压舌板将舌体向后下方推压，以长度75~100mm的芒针点刺悬雍垂两侧之咽后壁，每侧3~5点，少量出血，不留针。翳风，向咽部斜刺进针2寸，使麻胀感传至咽部。内关，向肘部斜刺，进针1.5寸，使麻胀感传至肘部，留针20分钟。

疗程：每日1次，10次为1个疗程，疗程间休息2日。

『推荐』

> 本方案适用于中风各期的一般假性球麻痹患者。[CRADE 2D]

7.2.2.6 靳三针疗法

此疗法是靳瑞教授在40余年临床实践的基础上，集历代针灸名家临床经验之精华，经反复、系统临床和实验研究总结创造出来的一种针灸流派，临床报道疗效较好。

取穴：脑三针（脑户、双侧脑空）和舌三针（上廉泉、上廉泉左右旁开各1寸）。

配穴：肝阳暴亢型配足临泣、太冲；风痰阻络型配风市、丰隆；痰热腑实型配曲池、丰隆；气虚血瘀型配足三里、三阴交；阴虚风动型配复溜、太溪。

针刺方法：所有穴位均按常规操作，针刺得气后，行平补平泻手法，配合电针治疗，电针参数选疏密波，频率为2/100Hz。

疗程：每日1次，20次为1个疗程。

『推荐』

推荐建议：本方案适用于中风各期的一般假性球麻痹患者。[CRADE 2D]

7.2.2.7 任督通调针刺法

此疗法是根据任督二脉在循行上与脑和咽喉有密切关系的特点，在二脉上选取腧穴为主治疗假性球麻痹的一种针刺方法，能有效改善中风后假性球麻痹患者吞咽障碍症状。

取穴：天突穴、廉泉穴、百会穴、脑户穴、哑门穴。

针刺方法：穴位局部皮肤用酒精棉球常规消毒。天突：仰靠坐位，取长度40mm的毫针，先直刺0.2寸，当针尖超过胸骨柄内缘后，即向下沿胸骨柄后缘、气管前缘缓慢向下刺入0.5~1寸，然后左手握住针柄缓慢捻转，待患者有闷胀感后慢慢捻转出针。廉泉：取坐位，用长度40mm的毫针，向舌根方向针刺，进针1~1.2寸，以轻手法提插3~5次，得气后将针尖提至皮下，再向咽部方向刺入0.5~0.8寸，以舌根、咽部有酸、痛、胀为佳，得气后留针30分钟，每10分钟行平补平泻手法1次。百会：取坐位，用长度25mm的毫针，平刺0.5~1寸，捻转2~3次，频率200次/分钟，得气后留针30分钟。脑户：取坐位，用长度25mm的毫针，平刺0.5~1寸，捻转2~3次，频率90~120次/分钟，得气后留针30分钟。哑门：取坐位，使头微前倾，项肌放松，用长度40mm的毫针，针尖向下颌方向，进针0.5~1寸，捻转泻法，频率90~120次/分钟，1分钟后出针。

疗程：每日1次，每周6次，每周休息1天，4周为1个疗程。

『推荐』

推荐建议：本方案适用于中风各期的一般假性球麻痹吞咽障碍患者。[CRADE 2D]

7.2.3 康复与中药治疗

建议参照相关诊疗常规进行，或咨询相关专业科室人员配合共同执行。

8 专家意见征集过程、结果汇总及处理

2014年3月20日总课题组在广安门医院召开《指南》统稿会，针对专家组提出的意见和建议对《指南》进行修改，结果如下：

意见汇总处理表

指南名称： 中风假性球麻痹 针灸临床实践指南	负责起草单位： 赵吉平	承办人： 刘保延	电话：84013147 共 页 第 页 2014年4月25日填写

序号	指南章条编号	意见内容	处理意见
1	干预与管理 1.3	针灸治疗疾病的原则部分：除了要写出针灸治疗该病症的原则外，还应归纳出治疗该病症的共性、核心内容，如写出针灸治疗的介入时机、治疗疗程等目前临床急需解答的主要临床问题	采纳了总课题组的意见。在针灸治疗总则部分增加了针灸治疗的介入时机、治疗疗程等重要临床内容
2	推荐方案	各推荐方案中，不需要再写出每个推荐方案（治疗方法）的原则，推荐方案包括简要说明、取穴、操作方法、疗程、注意事项这四部分。	采纳了总课题组的意见。原推荐方案缺少"简要说明"等内容，现予以补充和完善

续　表

序号	指南章条编号	意见内容	处理意见
3	推荐方案	注意事项只需要写该疗法（或方案）针对该疾病需要注意的内容，属于针灸治疗共性注意事项者则尽量不要写太多	采纳了总课题组的意见。原推荐方案缺少"简要说明"等内容，现予以补充和完善
4	推荐方案	术语和文字一定要规范，建议使用有关教材及相关针灸国家标准的名词术语	采纳了总课题组的意见。对《指南》的书写体例进行了规范和统一，个别用词不当之处给予修改
5	推荐方案	每条推荐方案后面增加形成推荐方案过程的说明	采纳了总课题组的意见。在推荐方案后增加"解释"内容，介绍推荐方案形成过程中所引用的文献及 GRADE 评价结果等内容

9　会议纪要

2014 年第一批针灸临床实践指南专家论证会会议纪要

时间：2014 年 3 月 6 日。

地点：中国中医科学院广安门医院。

参会人员：总课题组成员、北京市特聘评论专家及各课题组负责人及主要编写成员。

会议内容：① 5 个课题组分别汇报指南推荐方案编写情况；②与会专家提出意见和建议；③总课题组整理专家意见，进一步修改指南。

总课题组关于各指南统稿的要求：

（1）针灸治疗疾病的原则部分，除了要写出针灸治疗该病症的原则外，还应归纳出治疗该病症的共性、核心内容，如写出针灸治疗的介入时机、治疗疗程等目前临床急需解答的主要临床问题。

（2）各推荐方案中，不需要再写出每个推荐方案（治疗方法）的原则，推荐方案包括简要说明、取穴、操作方法、疗程、注意事项这四部分。

（3）注意事项只需要写该疗法（或方案）针对该疾病需要注意的内容，属于针灸治疗共性注意事项者则尽量不要写太多。

（4）术语和文字一定要规范，建议使用有关教材及相关针灸国家标准的名词术语。另外，热敏灸作为一特殊疗法，各组在操作上应统一，建议以赵吉平老师组所述有关文字为范本供其他各组参考。

（5）每条推荐方案后面增加形成推荐方案过程的说明。
